MW01265595

STROKE:
Signs You Will Have It

Treatments, Prevention, Risk Factors,
& Images

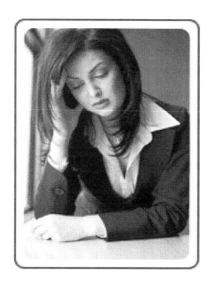

[ILLUSTRATED]

By James Lee Anderson

CONTENTS

INTRODUCTION TO STROKE

If you are like most Americans, you plan for your future. When you take a job, you examine its benefit plan. When you buy a home, you consider its location and condition so that your investment is safe. Today, more and more Americans are protecting their most important asset—their health. Are you?

Stroke ranks as the third leading killer in the United States. A stroke can be devastating to individuals and their families, robbing them of their independence. It is the most common cause of adult disability. Each year more than 795,000 Americans have a stroke, with about 160,000 dying from stroke-related causes.

Understanding Stroke

To understand stroke, it helps to know something about the brain. The brain controls our movements; stores our memories; and is the source of our thoughts, emotions, and language. The brain also controls many functions of the body, like breathing and digestion.

To work properly, your brain needs oxygen. Although your brain makes up only 2% of your body weight, it uses 20% of the oxygen you breathe. Your arteries deliver **oxygen-rich blood** to all parts of your brain.

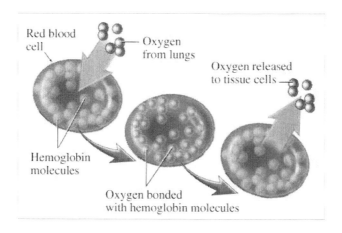

A **stroke** (or cerebrovascular accident) occurs when the blood supply to part of the brain is suddenly interrupted or when a blood vessel in the brain bursts, spilling blood into the spaces surrounding brain cells. In the same way that a person suffering a loss of blood flow to the heart is said to be having a heart attack, a person with a loss of blood flow to the brain or sudden bleeding in the brain can be said to be having a **"brain attack."**

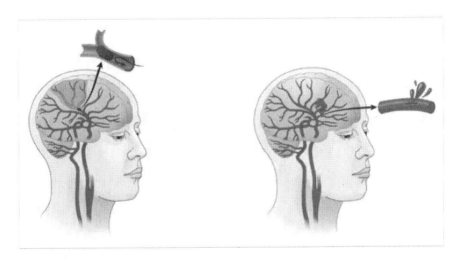

Left image: An ischemic stroke occurs when a blood vessel supplying the brain becomes blocked, as by a clot. **Right image:** A hemorrhagic stroke occurs when a blood vessel bursts, leaking blood into the brain.

Brain cells die when they no longer receive oxygen and nutrients from the blood or when they are damaged by sudden bleeding into or around the brain. *Ischemia* is the term used to describe the loss of oxygen and nutrients for brain cells when there is inadequate blood flow. Ischemia ultimately leads to *infarction*, the death of brain cells which are eventually replaced by a fluid-filled cavity (or *infarct*) in the injured brain.

There are two broad categories of stroke: those caused by a blockage of blood flow and those caused by bleeding. While not usually fatal, a **blockage of a blood vessel** in the brain or neck, called an *ischemic stroke*, is the most frequent cause of stroke and is responsible for about 80 percent of strokes. These blockages stem from three conditions: the formation of a clot within a blood vessel of the brain or neck, called *thrombosis*; the movement of a clot from another part of the body such as the heart to the neck or brain, called *embolism*; or a severe narrowing of an artery in or leading to the brain, called *stenosis*. **Bleeding into the brain** or the spaces surrounding the brain causes the second type of stroke, called *hemorrhagic stroke*.

Who Are Affected

Stroke causes more serious long-term disabilities than any other disease. Nearly three-quarters of all strokes occur in people over the age of 65 and the risk of having a stroke more than doubles each decade after the age of 55. For African Americans, stroke is more common and more deadly, even in young and middle-aged adults, than for any ethnic or other racial group in the United States. Learning about stroke can help you act in time to save a co-worker, friend, or relative. And making changes in your lifestyle can help you prevent stroke.

New treatments are available that greatly reduce the damage caused by a stroke. But you need to arrive at the hospital **within 60 minutes** after symptoms start to prevent disability. Knowing stroke symptoms, calling 911 immediately, and getting to a hospital are critical.

*"Someone in the United States has a stroke every **40 seconds**. Every **four minutes**, someone dies of stroke."*

Learn in detail about the types of stroke in the succeeding sections.

The following are different forms of stroke that are likely to affect people especially those who are at risk of getting this serious medical condition.

Ischemic Stroke

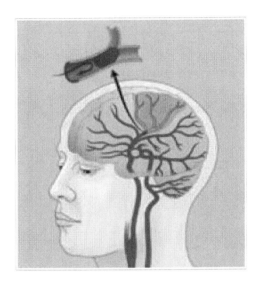

An **ischemic stroke** occurs when an artery supplying the brain with blood becomes blocked, suddenly decreasing or stopping blood flow and ultimately causing a brain infarction. This type of stroke accounts for approximately *80 percent* of all strokes. Blood clots are the most common cause of artery blockage and brain infarction. The process of clotting is necessary and beneficial throughout the body because it stops bleeding and allows repair of damaged areas of arteries or veins. However, when blood clots develop in the wrong place within an artery they can cause devastating injury by interfering with the normal flow of blood. Problems with clotting become more frequent as people age.

Blood clots can cause ischemia and infarction in two ways. A clot that forms in a part of the body other than the brain can travel through blood vessels and become wedged in a brain artery. This free-roaming clot is called an *embolus* and often forms in the heart. A stroke caused by an embolus is called an *embolic stroke*. The second kind of ischemic stroke, called a *thrombotic stroke*, is caused by *thrombosis*, the formation of a blood clot in one of the cerebral arteries that stays attached to the artery wall until it grows large enough to block blood flow.

Ischemic strokes can also be caused by **stenosis**, or a narrowing of the artery due to the buildup of *plaque* (a mixture of fatty substances, including *cholesterol* and other lipids) and blood clots along the artery wall. Stenosis can occur in large arteries and small arteries and is therefore called *large vessel disease* or *small vessel disease*, respectively. When a stroke occurs, due to small vessel disease, a very small infarction results; sometimes called a *lacunar infarction*, from the French word "lacune" meaning "gap" or "cavity." The most common blood vessel disease that causes stenosis is *atherosclerosis*. In atherosclerosis, deposits of plaque buildup along the inner walls of large and medium-sized arteries, causing thickening, hardening, and loss of elasticity of artery walls and decreased blood flow.

Hemorrhagic Stroke

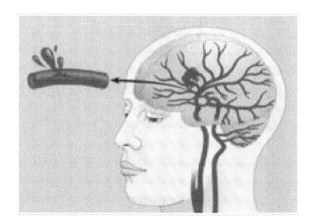

In a healthy, functioning brain, neurons do not come into direct contact with blood. The vital oxygen and nutrients the neurons need from the blood come to the neurons across the thin walls of the cerebral capillaries. The glia (nervous system cells that support and protect neurons) form a *blood-brain barrier*, an elaborate meshwork that surrounds blood vessels and capillaries and regulates which elements of the blood can pass through to the neurons.

When an artery in the brain **bursts**, blood spews out into the surrounding tissue and upsets not only the blood supply but the delicate chemical balance neurons require to function. This is called a **hemorrhagic stroke**. Such strokes account for approximately *20 percent* of all strokes.

Hemorrhage can occur in several ways. One common cause is a bleeding *aneurysm*, a weak or thin spot on an artery wall. Over time, these weak spots stretch or balloon out under high arterial pressure. The thin walls of these ballooning aneurysms can rupture and spill blood into the space surrounding brain cells.

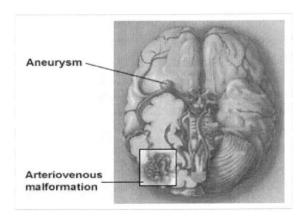

An aneurysm is a bulge in a blood vessel and an arteriovenous malformation is a tangled mass of thin-walled vessels. Both of these structures are associated with a risk of hemorrhagic stroke.

Hemorrhage also occurs when arterial walls break open. Plaque-encrusted artery walls eventually lose their elasticity and become brittle and thin, prone to cracking. *Hypertension*, or *high blood pressure*, increases the risk that a brittle artery wall will give way and release blood into the surrounding brain tissue.

A person with an ***arteriovenous malformation (AVM)*** also has an increased risk of hemorrhagic stroke. AVMs are a tangle of defective blood vessels and capillaries within the brain that have thin walls and can therefore rupture.

There are two types of hemorrhagic strokes:

- **Intracerebral hemorrhage** is the most common type of hemorrhagic stroke. It occurs when an artery in the brain bursts, flooding the surrounding tissue with blood.

- **Subarachnoid hemorrhage** is a less common type of hemorrhagic stroke. It refers to bleeding in the area between the brain and the thin tissues that cover it.

Transient Ischemic Attack (TIA)

A transient ischemic attack (TIA) is sometimes called a **"mini-stroke."** It is different from the major types of stroke because blood flow to the brain is blocked for only a short time—usually no more than 5 minutes.

It is important to know that

- A TIA is a warning sign of a future stroke.

- A TIA is a medical emergency, just like a major stroke.

- Strokes and TIAs require emergency care. **Call 9-1-1** right away if you feel signs of a stroke or see symptoms in someone around you.

- There is no way to know in the beginning whether symptoms are from a TIA or from a major type of stroke.

- Like ischemic strokes, blood clots often cause TIAs.

- More than a third of people who have a TIA end up having a major stroke within 1 year if they don't receive treatment, and 10%-15% will have a major stroke within 3 months of a TIA.

Recognizing and treating TIAs can reduce the risk of a major stroke. If you have a TIA, your health care team can find the cause and take steps to prevent a major stroke.

Recurrent Stroke

Recurrent stroke is frequent; about 25 percent of people who recover from their first stroke will have another stroke within 5 years. Recurrent stroke is a major contributor to stroke disability and death, with the risk of severe disability or death from stroke increasing with each stroke recurrence. The risk of a recurrent stroke is greatest right after a stroke, with the risk decreasing with time. About 3 percent of stroke patients will have another stroke within 30 days of their first stroke and one-third of recurrent strokes take place within 2 years of the first stroke.

CEREBRAL AMYLOID ANGIOPATHY

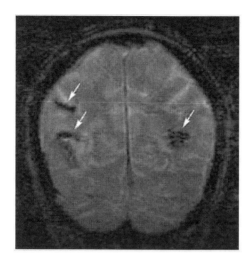

Cerebral amyloid angiopathy (CAA) refers to a buildup of protein deposits known as amyloid on the inside wall of blood vessels. It is a major contributing factor to *intracerebral hemorrhage* in older people and is sometimes associated with small ischemic infarctions and vascular cognitive impairment.

CAA is regarded as a disease of aging. It is rarely observed in individuals under age 50, but is seen in about 50 percent of individuals over age 90. The proportion of intracerebral hemorrhage cases in older people that are causally linked to CAA is unclear, but recent estimates place that number as high as 50 percent.

The buildup of amyloid inside blood vessels weakens the vessel wall and may lead to blood vessel rupture. In recent years, a poorly understood connection has emerged between CAA and Alzheimer's disease. Beta-amyloid - the toxic protein fragment that accumulates in clumps (called plaques) within the brain tissue of people with Alzheimer's disease - is a component of the amyloid deposits found in people with CAA. Moreover, Alzheimer's disease and CAA share similar genetic risk factors, such as the gene encoding apolipoprotein E (APOE). A variant of this gene known as e4 increases the risk of Alzheimer's disease and the risk of recurrent intracerebral hemorrhage.

Vascular Cognitive Impairment

Even in the absence of a clinically obvious stroke or TIA, impaired blood flow in the brain may eventually lead to **vascular cognitive impairment (VCI)**. At one extreme, VCI includes *vascular dementia, but it also refers to a gradual decline in mental function caused by multiple strokes, some silent, over time. It is often associated with a more diffuse small vessel disease, caused by narrowing of small-diameter blood vessels that supply limited territories within the brain. Clinically, VCI may resemble Alzheimer's disease (AD) and many older individuals with dementia meet the diagnostic criteria for both diseases. However, while AD primarily affects memory, VCI appears to primarily affect the brain's executive function-the ability to plan activities from getting dressed in the morning to negotiating a business deal.

Note: The word *vascular refers to vessels of the body, especially the arteries and veins, that carry blood and lymph.

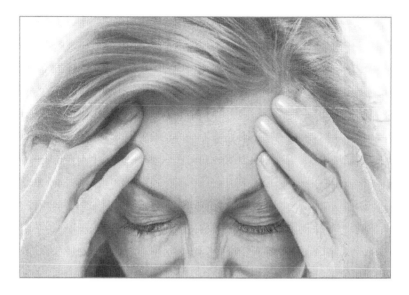

Sudden severe headache with no known cause is a stroke sign in men and women.

During a stroke, every minute counts! Fast treatment can reduce the brain damage that stroke can cause.

By knowing the signs and symptoms of stroke, you can be prepared to take quick action and perhaps save a life—maybe even your own.

Signs of Stroke in Men and Women

- Sudden **numbness** or weakness in the face, arm, or leg, especially on one side of the body.

- Sudden **confusion**, trouble speaking, or difficulty understanding speech.

- Sudden **trouble seeing** in one or both eyes.

- Sudden **trouble walking**, dizziness, loss of balance, or lack of coordination.

- Sudden **severe headache** with no known cause.

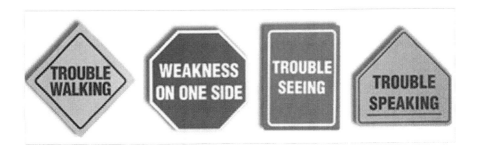

Call 9-1-1 immediately if you or someone else has any of these symptoms.

Acting F.A.S.T. is Key for Stroke

Acting F.A.S.T. can help stroke patients get the treatments they desperately need. The most effective stroke treatments are only available if the stroke is recognized and diagnosed within 3 hours of the first symptoms. Stroke patients may not be eligible for the most effective treatments if they don't arrive at the hospital in time.

If you think someone may be having a stroke, act F.A.S.T.[1] and do the following simple test:

F—Face: Ask the person to smile. Does one side of the face droop?

A—Arms: Ask the person to raise both arms. Does one arm drift downward?

S—Speech: Ask the person to repeat a simple phrase. Is their speech slurred or strange?

T—Time: If you observe any of these signs, call 9-1-1 immediately.

Note the time when any symptoms first appear. Some treatments for stroke only work if given in the first 3 hours after symptoms appear. Do not drive to the hospital or let someone else drive you. Call an ambulance so that medical personnel can begin life-saving treatment on the way to the emergency room.

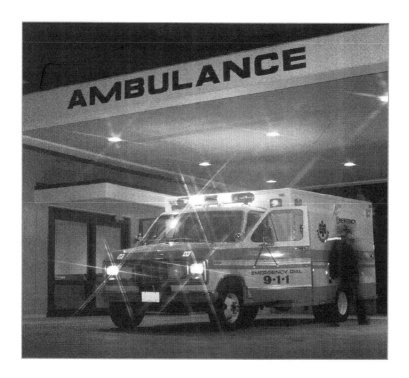

Treating a Transient Ischemic Attack

If your symptoms go away after a few minutes, you may have had a transient ischemic attack (TIA). Although brief, a TIA is a sign of a serious condition that will not go away without medical help. Tell your health care team about your symptoms right away.

Unfortunately, because TIAs clear up, many people ignore them. Don't be one of those people. Paying attention to a TIA can save your life.

Early Action Is Important for Stroke

Know the warning signs and symptoms of stroke so that you can act fast if you or someone you know might be having a stroke. The chances of survival are greater when emergency treatment begins quickly.

- In a 2005 survey, most respondents—93%—recognized sudden numbness on one side as a symptom of stroke. Only **38%** were aware of all major symptoms and knew to call 9-1-1 when someone was having a stroke.

- Patients who arrive at the emergency room within 3 hours of their first symptoms tend to have less disability 3 months after a stroke than those who received delayed care.

Stroke Survivors

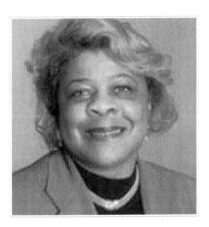

Stroke survivor Ruth Junious credits her quick recovery to a coworker who knew the warning signs. Photo courtesy of NIH/NINDS

When I walked into the locker room at work, I realized something was wrong. I couldn't speak. I tried to pick up my lock, but my right hand couldn't grab it." For Ruth Junious, the

sudden onset of a stroke was as bewildering as it was frightening.

"One of my co-workers noticed something was wrong and asked if I could write. With my left hand, I scribbled 911 on a piece of paper. Luckily, my friend knew the signs of stroke and got help. She called an ambulance, and I was rushed to the emergency room. The doctors ran some tests and put a drug into my IV. Within 10 minutes I could speak again."

The fact that her coworker knew the signs of stroke and understood the importance of urgent medical attention, may have saved Junious's life. Today, she understands much more about this disorder that occurs to more than 700,000 Americans each year— and is more common among African-Americans than any other racial or ethnic group in the United States.

"I didn't know a thing about stroke before I had one," she says. "Now, I make sure that all my family knows the signs of stroke, so they can get help if they need it."

Stroke occurs when blood flow to your brain is stopped, either by blockage of a blood vessel supplying the brain or rupture of a blood vessel that causes bleeding into the brain. And once you have a stroke, your chances of having another stroke are much greater. Many entertainers and other celebrities who have suffered a stroke go on to help warn others about the dangers, including such entertainers as Kirk Douglas and Della Reese, news broadcaster Mark McEwan, actress Julie Harris, and motivational speaker David Layton.

Preventing Stroke

"Until I had my stroke, I didn't do anything good for my health," says stroke survivor Ted Turner. *"I had high blood pressure, I was overweight, and I smoked. When bad things happen to people, they tend to think 'why me?' But, when I think about my stroke, I think*

'why not me?' I had all the risk factors and wasn't taking care of myself like I am now. I've learned a lot of important lessons from my stroke, which have caused me to change my eating habits, quit smoking, and really control my high blood pressure for the first time in my life. I hope people realize they can prevent stroke. It doesn't have to happen to them."

Like many stroke survivors, Turner knows the truth in the old saying that **"an ounce of prevention is worth a pound of cure."**

When Alma Shandling's husband Robert had a stroke, she knew just what to do.

"I could not speak," says Robert Shandling. *"All I knew was that she was my wife, and I reached over and took her hand. I couldn't remember the names of my grandchildren or my daughters. I was a complete blank."*

But Alma knew not only that it was a stroke, but that speed was of the essence. *"I said to him, 'You're having a stroke. Stay here. I'm going to call an ambulance,'"* Alma says. *"He made it to the hospital in about 25 minutes, and six days later he walked out of the hospital. I think that is a miracle; I really do."*

"Somehow, we have to get the hopeful message out that there is something you can do. It's not hopeless; you can do something," says John Marler, M.D., NINDS Associate Director for Clinical Trials. *"We've been able to develop a drug, t-PA, which you can inject in a vein, and it goes through the body, knows where the clot [causing the stroke] is, locks onto that clot, and dissolves it. And blood starts flowing again."*

Since about 80 percent of strokes involve a blood clot, t-PA has been a major advance in the treatment of strokes.

In fact, the risk of stroke in any given year is actually decreasing, notes Walter J. Koroshetz, M.D., NINDS Deputy Director. "Stroke rates have been decreasing since the 1960s and

'70s, and the annual risk of stroke death is still going down." Because stroke risk increases with age, as the population ages, total stroke incidence has not decreased. Progress in reducing risk is necessary just to keep up.

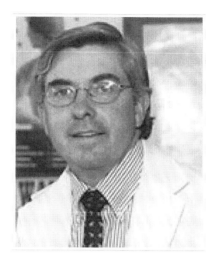

Walter Koroshetz, M.D., is Deputy Director of the National Institute of Neurological Disorder and Stroke (NINDS). Photo courtesy of NIH/NINDS

The challenge, Dr. Koroshetz adds, is to help people understand that some unhealthy lifestyle issues—high blood pressure, obesity, smoking—may prevent further declines in stroke rates. "Hypertension (high blood pressure) is the main risk factor for stroke," says Dr. Koroshetz. "And there is evidence that as you lower your cholesterol, stroke risk goes down. But the "epidemic" of obesity and sedentary lifestyle are acting against us. These are associated with high blood pressure and elevated cholesterol, atherosclerosis" (plaque buildup, causing narrowing in the arteries), and stroke risk.

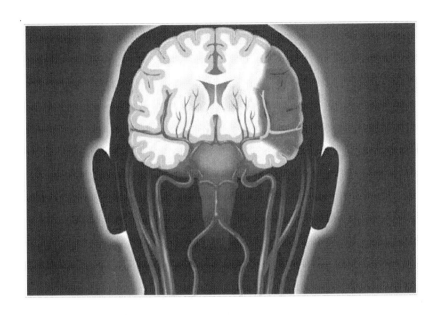

How is the Cause of Stroke Determined

Physicians have several diagnostic techniques and imaging tools to help diagnose the cause of stroke quickly and accurately. The first step in diagnosis is a short **neurological examination**. When a possible stroke patient arrives at a hospital, a health care professional, usually a doctor or nurse, will ask the patient or a companion what happened and when the symptoms began. **Blood tests**, an **electrocardiogram**, and a **brain scan**, such CT or MRI, will often be done. One test that helps doctors judge the severity of a stroke is the standardized National Institute of Health (NIH) Stroke Scale, developed by the National Institute of Neurological Disorder and Stroke (NINDS). Health care professionals use the NIH Stroke Scale to measure a patient's neurological deficits by asking the patient to answer questions and to perform several physical and mental tests. Other scales include the Glasgow Coma Scale, the Hunt and Hess Scale, the Modified Rankin Scale, and the Barthel Index.

Brain Imaging for the Diagnosis of Acute Stroke

Health care professionals also use a variety of imaging devices to evaluate stroke patients. The most widely used imaging procedure is the **computed tomography (CT) scan**. Also known as a CAT scan or computed axial tomography, CT creates a series of cross-sectional images of the head and brain. Because it is readily available at all hours at most major hospitals and produces images quickly, CT is the most commonly used diagnostic technique for acute stroke. CT also has unique diagnostic benefits. It will quickly rule out a hemorrhage, can occasionally show a tumor that might mimic a stroke, and may even show evidence of early infarction. Infarctions generally show up on a CT scan about 6 to 8 hours after the start of stroke symptoms.

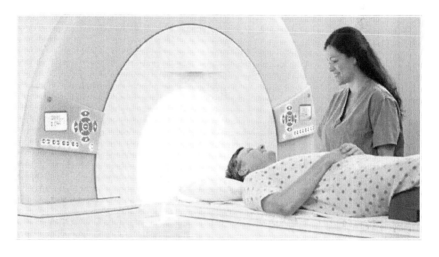

CT creates a series of cross-sectional images of the head and brain.

If a stroke is caused by hemorrhage, a CT scan show evidence of bleeding into the brain almost immediately after stroke symptoms appear. Hemorrhage is the primary reason for avoiding certain drug treatments for stroke, such as thrombolytic therapy, the only proven acute stroke therapy for ischemic stroke (*see* section on "What Stroke Therapies are Available?"). Thrombolytic therapy cannot be used until the doctor can confidently diagnose the patient as suffering from an ischemic stroke because this treatment might increase bleeding and could make a hemorrhagic stroke worse.

Another imaging device used for stroke patients is the **magnetic resonance imaging (MRI) scan**. MRI uses magnetic fields to detect subtle changes in brain tissue content. One effect of stroke is the slowing of water movement, called *diffusion*, through the damaged brain tissue. MRI can show this type of damage within the first hour after the stroke symptoms start. The benefit of MRI over a CT scan is more accurate and earlier diagnosis of infarction, especially for smaller strokes, while showing equivalent accuracy in determining when hemorrhage is present. MRI is more sensitive than CT for other types of brain disease, such as brain tumor, that might mimic a stroke. MRI cannot be performed in patients with certain types of metallic or electronic implants, such as pacemakers for the heart.

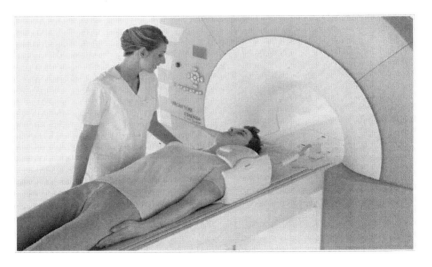

MRI scans are commonly used to check for damage to the brain and the brain's vasculature in people suspected of having a stroke.

Although increasingly used in the emergency diagnosis of stroke, MRI is not immediately available at all hours in most hospitals, where CT is used for acute stroke diagnosis. Also, MRI takes longer to perform than CT, and may not be performed if it would significantly delay treatment.

Other types of MRI scans, often used for the diagnosis of cerebrovascular disease and to predict the risk of stroke, are *magnetic resonance angiography (MRA)* and *functional magnetic resonance imaging (fMRI)*. Neurosurgeons use MRA to detect stenosis (blockage) of the brain arteries inside the skull by mapping flowing blood. Functional MRI uses a magnet to pick up signals from oxygenated blood and can show brain activity through increases in local blood flow. *Duplex Doppler ultrasound* and *arteriography* are two diagnostic imaging techniques used to decide if an individual would benefit from a surgical procedure called *carotid endarterectomy.* This surgery is used to remove fatty deposits from the carotid arteries and can help prevent stroke.

Doppler ultrasound is a painless, noninvasive test in which sound waves above the range of human hearing are sent into the neck. Echoes bounce off the moving blood and the tissue in the artery and can be formed into an image. Ultrasound is fast, painless, risk-free, and relatively inexpensive compared to MRA and arteriography, but it is not considered to be as accurate as arteriography. **Arteriography** is an X-ray of the carotid artery taken when a special dye is injected into the artery. The procedure carries its own small risk of causing a stroke and is costly to perform. The benefits of arteriography over MR techniques and ultrasound are that it is extremely reliable and still the best way to measure stenosis of the carotid arteries. Even so, significant advances are being made every day involving noninvasive imaging techniques such as fMRI.

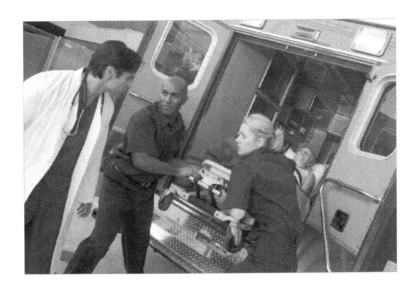

Emergency Treatment

Your emergency treatment starts in the ambulance. The emergency workers may take you to a specialized stroke center to ensure that you receive the quickest possible diagnosis and treatment.

At the hospital, health care providers will ask about your medical history and about the time your symptoms started. Brain scans will show what type of stroke you had. You may also work with a neurologist who treats brain disorders, a neurosurgeon that performs surgery on the brain, or a specialist in another area of medicine.

If you get to the hospital within 3 hours of the first symptoms of an ischemic stroke, a health care provider may give you a type of medicine called a thrombolytic (a "clot-busting" drug) to break up blood clots. Tissue plasminogen activator (tPA) is a thrombolytic.

Medications

Medicines that lower blood pressure and cholesterol can protect against atherosclerosis and reduce a person's risk of stroke. **Aspirin** and other blood-thinning medications have been used for years to reduce the risk of ischemic stroke in individuals with AF or prior stroke. Recent studies have helped refine the use of these drugs to maximize safety and efficacy. This section, however, begins with a discussion of what happens when prevention fails and a person requires emergency treatment for an acute ischemic stroke.

Thrombolytic Drugs

In treating acute ischemic stroke (acute meaning that the stroke has occurred within the past few hours), the immediate goal is to break apart the offending clot, a process known as thrombolysis. The body produces its own thrombolytic proteins, and some of these have been engineered into drugs. One, called **tissue plasminogen activator (tPA)**, had a proven track record for treating heart attacks. In the late 1980s, NINDS-funded investigators laid the plans for the first placebo-controlled trial of tPA to treat acute ischemic stroke. They knew from animal studies that irreversible brain injury is likely to occur if blood flow is not restored within the first few hours after ischemic stroke. Therefore, the NINDS tPA Study Group tested the drug within a three-hour time window. Compared to individuals given placebo, those given intravenous tPA were more likely to have minimal or no disability three months after treatment-a finding that persuaded the U.S. Food and Drug Administration to approve tPA for use against acute stroke. Trials in Europe and the U.S. subsequently confirmed those results. Recent studies attempt to identify individuals who may benefit even after three hours of stroke onset. In any case, more brain tissue will be saved the earlier the treatment is delivered.

A 1998 follow-up analysis of the NINDS trial found that, after their initial hospitalization, people who received tPA were less likely to require inpatient rehabilitation or nursing home care. The authors estimated that this lower dependency on long-term care would translate into a savings to the healthcare system of more than $4 million for every 1,000 individuals treated with tPA.

Because treatment with tPA interferes with blood clotting and has also been shown to increase leaking along the blood-brain barrier, it carries a risk of intracerebral hemorrhage. Therefore, it is not recommended for some people, such as those with a history of brain hemorrhage or significantly elevated blood pressure (greater than 185/110 mm Hg). The risk of tPA-induced hemorrhage increases over time from stroke onset, which has limited its use to the first three hours after stroke (where benefit was most clearly established in the U.S. trials).

Antiplatelet Drugs and Anticoagulants

Blood-thinning medications fall into two classes: antiplatelet drugs and anticoagulants. Antiplatelet drugs inhibit the activity of cells called platelets, which stick to damaged areas inside blood vessels and lay the foundation for blood clots. The most common antiplatelet drug is **aspirin**. Anticoagulants, such as **heparin** (produced by inflammatory cells in the body) and **warfarin** (found in plants and also known by the trade name Coumadin©), inhibit proteins in the blood that stimulate clotting.

Antiplatelet drugs and anticoagulants can help prevent a variety of potentially life-threatening conditions for which individuals with stroke are at risk, such as myocardial infarction, pulmonary embolism, and deep vein thrombosis-which are caused by clots in the heart, lungs and deep veins of the legs, respectively. In recent years, the value of these drugs in treating and preventing stroke itself has been more closely scrutinized.

One focus of this research has been to determine if there is any benefit in giving antiplatelet drugs or anticoagulants during an acute ischemic stroke, as an adjunct to tPA, or as an alternative for people ineligible to receive tPA. In an international trial coordinated by researchers in the United Kingdom in the late 1990s, individuals received aspirin, subcutaneous heparin injections, or neither treatment within 48 hours of an ischemic stroke. Aspirin significantly reduced the risk of a recurrent ischemic stroke at two weeks. A similar benefit from heparin was offset by an increased risk of hemorrhagic stroke. Around the same time, NINDS-funded researchers tested whether acute stroke could be treated with intravenous Org 10172, a form of heparin considered less likely to cause bleeding. This study, Trial of Org 10172 in Acute Stroke Treatment (TOAST), found that Org 10172 produced no significant benefit. The study authors also developed the TOAST criteria, a set of guidelines for classifying different subtypes of ischemic stroke that are now widely used in other studies.

Another issue is whether individuals at risk for ischemic stroke should be placed on a daily maintenance program of aspirin or anticoagulants. For many years, aspirin and warfarin were used as a means of stroke prevention in individuals with AF, but until recently, this practice was based more on anecdotal evidence than on scientific data. A systematic analysis of warfarin's benefits was especially important since it is an expensive drug and, like heparin, is associated with an increased risk of hemorrhagic stroke. The NINDS Boston Area Anticoagulation Trial for Atrial Fibrillation (BAATAF) and the Stroke Prevention in Atrial Fibrillation (SPAF) trials showed that daily warfarin is best for people with AF who are over age 65 or who have additional vascular risk factors. Daily aspirin provides adequate protection against stroke among young people with AF.

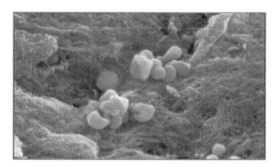

Platelets (magnified here thousands of times) home to damaged areas of blood vessels and contribute to the formation of clots. Antiplatelet drugs can help reduce the risk of ischemic stroke.

Two other NINDS-sponsored trials compared the effectiveness of daily warfarin and aspirin for individuals who did not have AF, but who had experienced a prior stroke-and thus were at risk for another. The Warfarin vs. Aspirin Recurrent Stroke Study (WARSS) showed that aspirin was as effective as warfarin in preventing recurrent stroke in people with no history of AF or other cardioembolic causes of stroke. The Warfarin-Aspirin Symptomatic Intracranial Disease (WASID) trial focused more narrowly on individuals with stenosis of arteries in the brain and was terminated early because of a high rate of adverse events in participants treated with warfarin. Both trials concluded that aspirin is equivalent to warfarin for reducing the risk of stroke in people without AF.

Medication for Subarachnoid Hemorrhage

The drug **nimodipine** is used to treat cerebral vasospasm, a complication that sometimes follows subarachnoid hemorrhage. This refers to a constriction of blood vessels in the brain that can significantly reduce blood flow, leading to ischemia and infarction. Although its precise origins are unclear, cerebral vasospasm is thought to be triggered in part by an influx of calcium into the smooth muscles that control blood vessel diameter. Nimodipine is a calcium antagonist, meaning that it works by blocking the entry of calcium into cells. Nimodipine has been shown to reduce infarction and improve outcome in individuals with subarachnoid hemorrhage.

Robert, a 74 year-old retiree...

...had just stepped inside after watering the lawn when he suddenly felt odd. He tried to speak to his wife, Alma, but realized that he couldn't. He held her hand and stared at her. He didn't know what was happening to him, but fortunately, she did.

As an avid reader of health information, Alma immediately recognized that Robert was having a stroke. She dialed 911, and about 30 minutes later, Robert was in an emergency room. Doctors quickly took pictures of Robert's brain using a CT scan and determined that his stroke was ischemic in nature. In other words, a clot was blocking the flow of blood to vital brain areas, including the speech center. They also determined that Robert was a good candidate for tPA, a clot-busting drug that had been approved for use against acute ischemic stroke by the Food and Drug Administration in 1996, just four years earlier.

While the doctors administered tPA intravenously, they asked Robert a series of simple questions to test his ability to think and speak - questions like "Do you know where you are?" and "Can you name your wife and children? Your grandchildren?" At first, his speech continued to fail him, but after a few minutes, he was answering every question. He was released from the hospital 6 days later, and after some speech therapy, he was soon reading to his grandchildren again.

During Robert's treatment and evaluation at the hospital, doctors discovered that he had atrial fibrillation (AF), which is an abnormal heart rhythm and a risk factor for stroke. He now takes warfarin, a medication that inhibits blood clotting and has proven effective for reducing the risk of stroke in people with AF and other stroke risk factors. He hasn't experienced any more strokes.

Robert and Alma have seven grandchildren and one great-granddaughter. Robert continues to enjoy reading to the youngest ones.

Surgeries and Other Procedures

Surgery is sometimes used to clear the congested blood vessels that cause ischemic stroke or to repair the vascular abnormalities that contribute to hemorrhagic stroke.

A surgery called **carotid endarterectomy** involves removing plaque to widen the carotids, a pair of arteries that ascend each side of the neck and are the main suppliers of blood to the brain. Stenosis that narrows a carotid artery by more than 50 percent is considered clinically significant. In some cases, carotid stenosis is first detected after a person experiences a stroke or other symptoms, such as a TIA. It is also sometimes detected in the absence of symptoms, as when a physician presses a stethoscope to the neck and hears a bruit- a sound made by blood flowing past an obstruction. The presence of carotid stenosis can be confirmed by angiography or Doppler ultrasound.

Data from NINDS-funded research show that the risk of ischemic stroke from clinically significant asymptomatic carotid stenosis is about two to three percent per year (meaning that out of 100 individuals with this condition, two or three will have a stroke each year). The risk of ischemic stroke from clinically significant symptomatic carotid stenosis is much higher-about 25 percent during the first two years following the appearance of symptoms.

Jim, a 58 year-old businessman...

...was spending a Saturday morning preparing for a church retreat, when he was struck by a headache and a strange feeling in his throat. Thinking maybe he had strep throat, he asked his wife Judy to drive him to an urgent care center. He felt too drained to drive himself.

The urgent care doctor quickly recognized that Jim was having a stroke, and sent the couple to the nearest emergency department. On the way, Jim's speech slurred, the right side of his face drooped, and the limbs on his right side grew heavy.

At the hospital, a CT scan indicated damage to the left side of Jim's brainstem. This is the part of the brain that connects to the spinal cord, so the CT findings fit with the weakness Jim had on the right side of his body. The stroke was caused by a blood clot, but for medical reasons, Jim was not eligible for the clot-busting drug tPA.

Jim stayed under observation in intensive care for 3 days. When he was released, he could not walk or use his right hand, so he spent a month at an inpatient rehabilitation center, where he received *physical and occupational therapy. When he left the center, he had little function in his right hand, but he was able to walk with a four-pronged cane.*

It has been more than 7 years since Jim's stroke. He exercises regularly and can walk unassisted, but he still has trouble with his right hand. By participating in clinical research, he is receiving an experimental treatment called constraint-induced movement therapy. This involves wearing a large mitt that limits movement of his left hand, forcing him to use his right hand for daily activities. Researchers expect the therapy to be most effective within the first year after a stroke, but Jim has noticed some improvement. Although writing and eating remain easier with his left hand, he can do both with his right. He continues to be very active at church and in his community.

NINDS-supported research has compared the benefits of standard medical therapy alone (treatment with aspirin, blood pressure-lowering drugs, and cholesterol-lowering drugs) with standard medical therapy plus endarterectomy for both types of carotid stenosis. The Asymptomatic Carotid Atherosclerosis Study (ACAS) found that endarterectomy cut the risk of stroke in half among individuals with asymptomatic carotid stenosis of 60 percent or greater. The NINDS North American Symptomatic Carotid Endarterectomy Trial (NASCET) found major benefits for individuals with symptomatic carotid stenosis of 70 percent or greater. Their risk of stroke over a two-year period was cut to less than 10 percent.

Endarterectomy itself is associated with a small risk of stroke because the disruption of plaque during the procedure can send emboli into the bloodstream, or cause a clot at the site of surgery. NINDS supports the investigation of an alternative procedure known as **carotid artery stenting**, which involves inserting a stent (a tube-like device that is made of mesh-like material) into the carotid artery. The stent is compressed until the radiologist threads it into position, and is then expanded to mechanically widen the artery. It is also equipped with a downstream "umbrella" to catch dislodged plaque. The Carotid Revascularization Endarterectomy vs. Stenting Trial (CREST) is designed to compare these two procedures in individuals with symptomatic carotid stenosis.

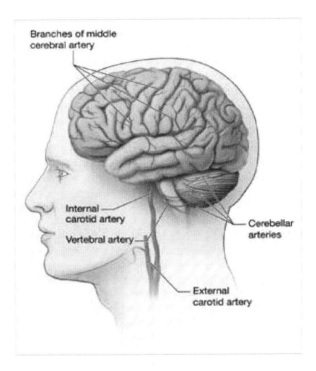

The carotid and vertebral arteries ascend through the neck and divide into branches that supply blood to different parts of the brain.

Several techniques are used to eliminate the vascular abnormalities linked to hemorrhagic stroke, or at least to reduce the risk that they will rupture. Arteriovenous malformations (AVMs) can be surgically removed through a procedure known as surgical resection. They can also be treated non-invasively (without the need to cut into the skull) using radiosurgery or embolization. **Radiosurgery** involves directing a beam of radiation at the AVM, while **embolization** involves injecting artificial emboli (usually made of foam) into the AVM to block it off from its parent vessel.

Clipping and coiling are procedures used to treat intracerebral aneurysms. Clipping involves opening the skull and placing a clip near the aneurysm, to separate it from its parent blood vessel. In endovascular coiling, a wire topped with a detachable coil is inserted into a leg artery and threaded into the aneurysm. Once in place, the coil is released into the aneurysm, where it stimulates blood clotting and strengthens the blood vessel wall. Stents are also used in some cases to divert blood flow away from an aneurysm. The carotid and vertebral arteries ascend through the neck and divide into branches that supply blood to different parts of the brain.

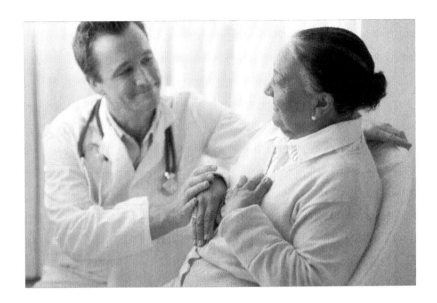

If you have had a, you are at high risk for another stroke:

- 1 of 4 stroke survivors has another stroke within 5 years.

- The risk of stroke within 90 days of a TIA may be as high as 17%, with the greatest risk during the first week.

That's why it's important to treat the underlying causes of stroke, including heart disease, high blood pressure, atrial fibrillation (fast, irregular heartbeat), high cholesterol, and diabetes. Your doctor may give you medications or tell you to change your diet, exercise, or adopt other healthy lifestyle habits. Surgery may also be helpful in some cases.

The long-term outcomes after a stroke vary considerably and depend partly on the type of stroke and the age of the affected person. Although most stroke survivors regain their functional independence, 15 to 30 percent will have a permanent physical disability. Some will experience a permanent decline in cognitive function known as post-stroke or vascular dementia. Unfortunately, many stroke survivors face a danger of recurrent stroke in the future. About 20 to 25 percent of people who experience a first-ever stroke between ages 40 and 69 will have another stroke within five years. Finding treatments to help prevent stroke in this high-risk group is a major focus of NINDS-supported research.

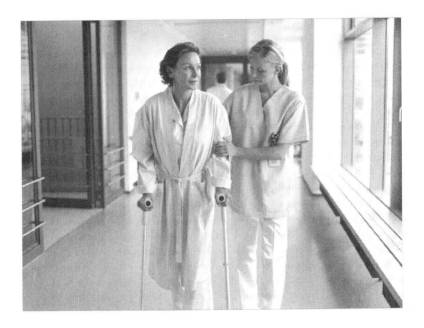

In the United States more than 795,000 people suffer a stroke each year, and approximately two-thirds of these individuals survive and require rehabilitation. The goals of rehabilitation are to help survivors become as independent as possible and to attain the best possible quality of life. Even though rehabilitation does not "cure" the effects of stroke in that it does not reverse brain damage, rehabilitation can substantially help people achieve the best possible long-term outcome.

What Is Post-Stroke Rehabilitation

Rehabilitation helps stroke survivors relearn skills that are lost when part of the brain is damaged. For example, these skills can include coordinating leg movements in order to walk or carrying out the steps involved in any complex activity. Rehabilitation also teaches survivors new ways of performing tasks to circumvent or compensate for any residual disabilities. Individuals may need to learn how to bathe and dress using only one hand, or how to communicate effectively when their ability to use language has been compromised. There is a strong consensus among rehabilitation experts that the most important element in any rehabilitation program is carefully directed, well-focused, repetitive practice—the same kind of practice used by all people when they learn a new skill, such as playing the piano or pitching a baseball.

Rehabilitative therapy begins in the *acute-care hospital* after the person's overall condition has been stabilized, often within 24 to 48 hours after the stroke. The first steps involve promoting independent movement because many individuals are paralyzed or seriously weakened. Patients are prompted to change positions frequently while lying in bed and to engage in **passive or active range of motion exercises** to strengthen their stroke-impaired limbs. ("Passive" range-of-motion exercises are those in which the therapist actively helps the patient move a limb repeatedly, whereas "active" exercises are performed by the patient with no physical assistance from the therapist.) Depending on many factors—including the extent of the initial injury—patients may progress from sitting up and being moved between the bed and a chair to standing, bearing their own weight, and walking, with or without assistance. Rehabilitation nurses and therapists help patients who are able to perform progressively more complex and demanding tasks, such as bathing, dressing, and using a toilet, and they encourage patients to begin using their stroke-impaired limbs while engaging in those tasks. Beginning to reacquire the ability to carry out these basic activities of daily living represents the first stage in a stroke survivor's return to independence.

For some stroke survivors, rehabilitation will be an ongoing process to maintain and refine skills and could involve working with specialists for months or years after the stroke.

What Disabilities Can Result From a Stroke

The types and degrees of disability that follow a stroke depend upon which area of the brain is damaged. Generally, stroke can

35

cause five types of disabilities: paralysis or problems controlling movement; sensory disturbances including pain; problems using or understanding language; problems with thinking and memory; and emotional disturbances.

Paralysis or problems controlling movement (motor control)

Paralysis is one of the most common disabilities resulting from stroke. The paralysis is usually on the side of the body opposite the side of the brain damaged by stroke, and may affect the face, an arm, a leg, or the entire side of the body. This one-sided paralysis is called *hemiplegia* (one-sided weakness is called *hemiparesis*). Stroke patients with hemiparesis or hemiplegia may have difficulty with everyday activities such as walking or grasping objects. Some stroke patients have problems with swallowing, called *dysphagia*, due to damage to the part of the brain that controls the muscles for swallowing. Damage to a lower part of the brain, the cerebellum, can affect the body's ability to coordinate movement, a disability called *ataxia*, leading to problems with body posture, walking, and balance.

Sensory disturbances including pain

Stroke patients may lose the ability to feel touch, pain, temperature, or position. Sensory deficits also may hinder the ability to recognize objects that patients are holding and can even be severe enough to cause loss of recognition of one's own limb. Some stroke patients experience pain, numbness or odd sensations of tingling or prickling in paralyzed or weakened limbs, a symptom known as *paresthesias*.

The loss of urinary continence is fairly common immediately after a stroke and often results from a combination of sensory and motor deficits. Stroke survivors may lose the ability to sense the need to urinate or the ability to control bladder muscles. Some may lack enough mobility to reach a toilet in time. Loss of bowel control or constipation also may occur. Permanent incontinence after a stroke is uncommon, but even a temporary loss of bowel or bladder control can be emotionally difficult for stroke survivors.

Stroke survivors frequently have a variety of chronic pain syndromes resulting from stroke-induced damage to the nervous system (neuropathic pain). In some stroke patients, pathways for sensation in the brain are damaged, causing the transmission of false signals that result in the sensation of pain in a limb or side of the body that has the sensory deficit. The most common of these pain syndromes is called "thalamic pain syndrome" (caused by a stroke to the thalamus, which processes sensory information from the body to the brain), which can be difficult to treat even with medications. Finally, some pain that occurs after stroke is not due to nervous system damage, but rather to mechanical problems caused by the weakness from the stroke. Patients who have a seriously weakened or paralyzed arm commonly experience moderate to severe pain that radiates outward from the shoulder. Most often, the pain results from lack of movement in a joint that has been immobilized for a prolonged period of time (such as having your arm or shoulder in a cast for weeks) and the tendons and ligaments around the joint become fixed in one position. This is commonly called a "frozen" joint; "passive" movement (the joint is gently moved or flexed by a therapist or caregiver rather than by the individual) at the joint in a paralyzed limb is essential to prevent painful "freezing" and to allow easy movement if and when voluntary motor strength returns.

Problems using or understanding language (aphasia)

At least one-fourth of all stroke survivors experience language impairments, involving the ability to speak, write, and understand spoken and written language. A stroke-induced injury to any of the brain's language-control centers can severely impair verbal communication. The dominant centers for language are in the left side of the brain for right-handed individuals and many left-handers as well. Damage to a language center located on the dominant side of the brain, known as Broca's area, causes *expressive aphasia*. People with this type of aphasia have difficulty conveying their thoughts through words or writing. They lose the ability to speak the words they are thinking and to put words together in coherent, grammatically correct sentences. In contrast, damage to a language center located in a rear portion of the brain, called Wernicke's area, results in *receptive aphasia*. People with this condition have difficulty understanding spoken or written language and often have incoherent speech. Although they can form grammatically correct sentences, their utterances are often devoid of meaning. The most severe form of aphasia, *global aphasia*, is caused by extensive damage to several areas of the brain involved in language function. People with global aphasia lose nearly all their linguistic abilities; they cannot understand language or use it to convey thought.

Problems with thinking and memory

Stroke can cause damage to parts of the brain responsible for memory, learning, and awareness. Stroke survivors may have dramatically shortened attention spans or may experience deficits in short-term memory. Individuals also may lose their ability to make plans, comprehend meaning, learn new tasks, or engage in other complex mental activities. Two fairly common deficits resulting from stroke are *anosognosia*, an inability to acknowledge the reality of the physical impairments resulting from stroke, and *neglect*, the loss of the ability to respond to objects or sensory stimuli located on the stroke-impaired side. Stroke survivors who develop *apraxia* (loss of ability to carry out a learned purposeful movement) cannot plan the steps involved in a complex task and act on them in the proper sequence. Stroke survivors with apraxia also may have problems following a set of instructions. Apraxia appears to be caused by a disruption of the subtle connections that exist between thought and action.

Emotional disturbances

Many people who survive a stroke feel fear, anxiety, frustration, anger, sadness, and a sense of grief for their physical and mental losses. These feelings are a natural response to the psychological trauma of stroke. Some emotional disturbances and personality

38

changes are caused by the physical effects of brain damage. Clinical depression, which is a sense of hopelessness that disrupts an individual's ability to function, appears to be the emotional disorder most commonly experienced by stroke survivors. Signs of clinical depression include sleep disturbances, a radical change in eating patterns that may lead to sudden weight loss or gain, lethargy, social withdrawal, irritability, fatigue, self-loathing, and suicidal thoughts. Post-stroke depression can be treated with antidepressant medications and psychological counseling.

What Medical Professionals Specialize In Post-Stroke Rehabilitation

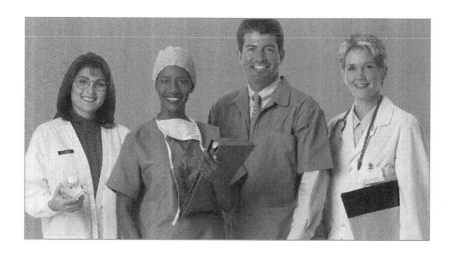

Post-stroke rehabilitation involves physicians; rehabilitation nurses; physical, occupational, recreational, speech-language, and vocational therapists; and mental health professionals.

Physicians

Physicians have the primary responsibility for **managing and coordinating the long-term care** of stroke survivors, including recommending which rehabilitation programs will best address individual needs. Physicians also are responsible for caring for the stroke survivor's general health and providing guidance aimed at preventing a second stroke, such as controlling high blood pressure or diabetes and eliminating risk factors such as cigarette smoking, excessive weight, a high-cholesterol diet, and high alcohol consumption.

Neurologists usually lead acute-care stroke teams and direct patient care during hospitalization. They sometimes participate on the long-term rehabilitation team. Other subspecialists often lead the rehabilitation stage of care, especially *physiatrists*, who specialize in physical medicine and rehabilitation.

Rehabilitation nurses

Nurses specializing in rehabilitation help survivors relearn how to carry out the basic **activities of daily living**. They also educate survivors about routine health care, such as how to follow a medication schedule, how to care for the skin, how to move out of a bed and into a wheelchair, and special needs for people with diabetes. Rehabilitation nurses also work with survivors to reduce risk factors that may lead to a second stroke, and provide training for caregivers.

Nurses are closely involved in helping stroke survivors manage personal care issues, such as bathing and controlling incontinence. Most stroke survivors regain their ability to maintain continence, often with the help of strategies learned during rehabilitation. These strategies include strengthening pelvic muscles through special exercises and following a timed voiding schedule. If problems with incontinence continue, nurses can help caregivers learn to insert and manage catheters and to take special hygienic measures to prevent other incontinence-related health problems from developing.

Physical therapists

Physical therapists specialize in treating disabilities related to **motor and sensory impairments**. They are trained in all aspects of anatomy and physiology related to normal function, with an emphasis on movement. They assess the stroke survivor's strength, endurance, range of motion, gait abnormalities, and sensory deficits to design individualized rehabilitation programs aimed at regaining control over motor functions.

Physical therapists help survivors regain the use of stroke-impaired limbs, teach compensatory strategies to reduce the effect of remaining deficits, and establish ongoing exercise programs to help people retain their newly learned skills. Disabled people tend to avoid using impaired limbs, a behavior called *learned non-use*. However, the repetitive use of impaired limbs encourages brain *plasticity* and helps reduce disabilities.

Strategies used by physical therapists to encourage the use of impaired limbs include selective sensory stimulation such as tapping or stroking, active and passive range-of-motion exercises, and temporary restraint of healthy limbs while practicing motor tasks.

In general, physical therapy emphasizes practicing isolated movements, repeatedly changing from one kind of movement to another, and rehearsing complex movements that require a great deal of coordination and balance, such as walking up or down stairs or moving safely between obstacles. People too weak to bear their own weight can still practice repetitive movements during hydrotherapy (in which water provides sensory stimulation as well as weight support) or while being partially supported by a harness. A recent trend in physical therapy emphasizes the effectiveness of engaging in goal-directed activities, such as playing games, to promote coordination. Physical therapists frequently employ selective sensory stimulation to encourage use of impaired limbs and to help survivors with neglect regain awareness of stimuli on the neglected side of the body.

41

Occupational and recreational therapists

Like physical therapists, occupational therapists are concerned with improving motor and sensory abilities, and ensuring patient safety in the post-stroke period. They help survivors relearn skills needed for performing **self-directed activities** (also called occupations) such as personal grooming, preparing meals, and housecleaning. Therapists can teach some survivors how to adapt to driving and provide on-road training. They often teach people to divide a complex activity into its component parts, practice each part, and then perform the whole sequence of actions. This strategy can improve coordination and may help people with apraxia relearn how to carry out planned actions.

Occupational therapists also teach people how to develop compensatory strategies and change elements of their environment that limit activities of daily living. For example, people with the use of only one hand can substitute hook and loop fasteners (such as Velcro) for buttons on clothing. Occupational therapists also help people make changes in their homes to increase safety, remove barriers, and facilitate physical functioning, such as installing grab bars in bathrooms.

Recreational therapists help people with a variety of disabilities to develop and use their leisure time to enhance their health, independence, and quality of life.

Speech-language pathologists

Speech-language pathologists help stroke survivors with aphasia relearn how to use **language or develop alternative means of communication**. They also help people improve their ability to swallow, and they work with patients to develop problem-solving and social skills needed to cope with the after-effects of a stroke.

Many specialized therapeutic techniques have been developed to assist people with aphasia. Some forms of short-term therapy can improve comprehension rapidly. Intensive exercises such as

42

repeating the therapist's words, practicing following directions, and doing reading or writing exercises form the cornerstone of language rehabilitation. Conversational coaching and rehearsal, as well as the development of prompts or cues to help people remember specific words, are sometimes beneficial. Speech-language pathologists also help stroke survivors develop strategies for circumventing language disabilities. These strategies can include the use of symbol boards or sign language. Recent advances in computer technology have spurred the development of new types of equipment to enhance communication.

Speech-language pathologists use special types of imaging techniques to study swallowing patterns of stroke survivors and identify the exact source of their impairment. Difficulties with swallowing have many possible causes, including a delayed swallowing reflex, an inability to manipulate food with the tongue, or an inability to detect food remaining lodged in the cheeks after swallowing. When the cause has been pinpointed, speech-language pathologists work with the individual to devise strategies to overcome or minimize the deficit. Sometimes, simply changing body position and improving posture during eating can bring about improvement. The texture of foods can be modified to make swallowing easier; for example, thin liquids, which often cause choking, can be thickened. Changing eating habits by taking small bites and chewing slowly can also help alleviate dysphagia.

Vocational therapists

Approximately one-fourth of all strokes occur in people between the ages of 45 and 65. For most people in this age group, returning to work is a major concern. Vocational therapists perform many of the same functions that ordinary career counselors do. They can help people with residual disabilities identify **vocational strengths** and develop résumés that highlight those strengths. They also can help identify potential employers, assist in specific job searches, and provide referrals to stroke vocational rehabilitation agencies.

Most important, vocational therapists educate disabled individuals about their **rights and protections** as defined by the Americans with Disabilities Act of 1990. This law requires employers to make *"reasonable accommodations"* for disabled employees. Vocational therapists frequently act as mediators between employers and employees to negotiate the provision of reasonable accommodations in the workplace.

When Can a Stroke Patient Get Rehabilitation

Rehabilitation should begin as soon as a stroke patient is stable, sometimes within 24 to 48 hours after a stroke. This first stage of rehabilitation can occur within an acute-care hospital; however, it is very dependent on the unique circumstances of the individual patient.

Recently, in the largest stroke rehabilitation study in the United States, researchers compared two common techniques to help stroke patients improve their walking. Both methods—training on a body-weight supported treadmill or working on strength and balance exercises at home with a physical therapist—resulted in equal improvements in the individual's ability to walk by the end of one year. Researchers found that functional improvements could be seen as late as one year after the stroke, which goes against the conventional wisdom that most recovery is complete by 6 months. The trial showed that 52 percent of the participants made significant improvements in walking, everyday function and quality of life, regardless of how severe their impairment was, or whether they started the training at 2 or 6 months after the stroke..

Where Can a Stroke Patient Get Rehabilitation

At the time of discharge from the hospital, the stroke patient and family coordinate with hospital social workers to locate a suitable living arrangement. Many stroke survivors return home, but some move into some type of medical facility.

Inpatient rehabilitation units

Inpatient facilities may be freestanding or part of larger hospital complexes. Patients stay in the facility, usually for 2 to 3 weeks, and engage in a coordinated, intensive program of rehabilitation. Such programs often involve at least 3 hours of active therapy a day, 5 or 6 days a week. Inpatient facilities offer a comprehensive range of medical services, including full-time physician supervision and access to the full range of therapists specializing in post-stroke rehabilitation.

Outpatient units

Outpatient facilities are often part of a larger hospital complex and provide access to physicians and the full range of therapists specializing in stroke rehabilitation. Patients typically spend several hours, often 3 days each week, at the facility taking part in coordinated therapy sessions and return home at night. Comprehensive outpatient facilities frequently offer treatment programs as intense as those of inpatient facilities, but they also can offer less demanding regimens, depending on the patient's physical capacity.

Nursing facilities

Rehabilitative services available at nursing facilities are more variable than are those at inpatient and outpatient units. Skilled nursing facilities usually place a greater emphasis on rehabilitation, whereas traditional nursing homes emphasize residential care. In addition, fewer hours of therapy are offered compared to outpatient and inpatient rehabilitation units.

Home-based rehabilitation programs

Home rehabilitation allows for great flexibility so that patients can tailor their program of rehabilitation and follow individual schedules. Stroke survivors may participate in an intensive level of therapy several hours per week or follow a less demanding regimen. These arrangements are often best suited for people who require treatment by only one type of rehabilitation therapist. Patients dependent on Medicare coverage for their rehabilitation must meet Medicare's "homebound" requirements to qualify for such services; at this time lack of transportation is not a valid reason for home therapy. The major disadvantage of home-based rehabilitation programs is the lack of specialized equipment. However, undergoing treatment at home gives people the advantage of practicing skills and developing compensatory strategies in the context of their own living environment. In the recent stroke rehabilitation trial, intensive balance and strength rehabilitation in the home was equivalent to treadmill training at a rehabilitation facility in improving walking.

What Research Is Being Done

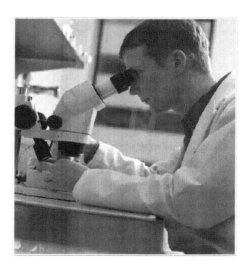

The National Institute of Neurological Disorders and Stroke (NINDS), a component of the U.S. National Institutes of Health (NIH), has primary responsibility for sponsoring research on disorders of the brain and nervous system, including the **acute phase of stroke** and the **restoration of function after stroke**. The

NIH's *Eunice Kennedy Shriver* National Institute of Child Health and Human Development, through its National Center for Medical Rehabilitation Research, funds work on mechanisms of restoration and repair after stroke, as well as development of new approaches to rehabilitation and evaluation of outcomes. Most of the NIH-funded work on **diagnosis and treatment of dysphagia** is through the National Institute on Deafness and Other Communication Disorders. The National Institute of Biomedical Imaging and Bioengineering collaborates with NINDS and NICHD in developing new instrumentation for stroke treatment and rehabilitation. The National Eye Institute funds work directed at **restoration of vision** and rehabilitation for individuals with impaired or low vision that may be due to vascular disease or stroke.

The NINDS supports research on ways to enhance **repair and regeneration of the central nervous system**. Scientists funded by the NINDS are studying how the brain responds to experience or adapts to injury by reorganizing its functions (plasticity)—using noninvasive imaging technologies to map patterns of biological activity inside the brain. Other NINDS-sponsored scientists are looking at brain reorganization after stroke and determining whether specific rehabilitative techniques, such as **constraint-induced movement therapy** and **transcranial magnetic stimulation**, can stimulate brain plasticity, thereby improving motor function and decreasing disability. Other scientists are experimenting with implantation of neural stem cells, to see if these cells may be able to replace the cells that died as a result of a stroke.

RISK FACTORS FOR STROKE

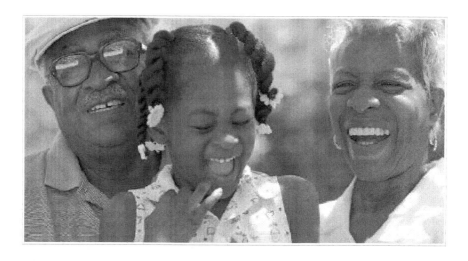

Who Is At Risk for Stroke

Some people are at a higher risk for stroke than others. Unmodifiable risk factors include age, gender, race/ethnicity, and stroke family history. In contrast, other risk factors for stroke, like high blood pressure or cigarette smoking, can be changed or controlled by the person at risk.

Unmodifiable Risk Factors

It is a myth that stroke occurs only in elderly adults. In actuality, stroke strikes all **age** groups, from fetuses still in the womb to centenarians. However, it is true that *older people* have a higher risk for stroke than the general population and that the risk for stroke increases with age. For every decade after the age of 55, the risk of stroke doubles, and two-thirds of all strokes occur in people over 65 years old. People over 65 also have a seven-fold greater risk of dying from stroke than the general population. And the incidence of stroke is increasing proportionately with the increase in the elderly population. When the baby boomers move into the over-65 age group, stroke and other diseases will take on even greater significance in the health care field.

Gender also plays a role in risk for stroke. *Men* have a higher risk for stroke, but more women die from stroke. The stroke risk for men is 1.25 times that for women. But men do not live as long as women, so men are usually younger when they have their strokes and therefore have a higher rate of survival than women. In other words, even though women have fewer strokes than men, women are generally older when they have their strokes and are more likely to die from them.

Stroke seems to run in some families. Several factors might contribute to **familial** stroke risk. Members of a family might have a genetic tendency for stroke risk factors, such as an inherited predisposition for hypertension or diabetes. The influence of a common lifestyle among family members could also contribute to familial stroke.

The risk for stroke varies among different **ethnic and racial** groups. The incidence of stroke among *African-Americans* is almost double that of white Americans, and twice as many African-Americans who have a stroke die from the event compared to white Americans. African-Americans between the ages of 45 and 55 have four to five times the stroke death rate of whites. After age 55 the stroke mortality rate for whites increases and is equal to that of African-Americans.

Compared to white Americans, African-Americans have a higher incidence of stroke risk factors, including high blood pressure and cigarette smoking. African-Americans also have a higher incidence and prevalence of some genetic diseases, such as diabetes and sickle cell anemia, which predispose them to stroke.

Hispanics and Native Americans have stroke incidence and mortality rates more similar to those of white Americans. In Asian-Americans stroke incidence and mortality rates are also similar to those in white Americans, even though Asians in Japan, China, and other countries of the Far East have significantly higher stroke incidence and mortality rates than white Americans. This suggests that environment and lifestyle factors play a large role in stroke risk.

The "Stroke Belt"

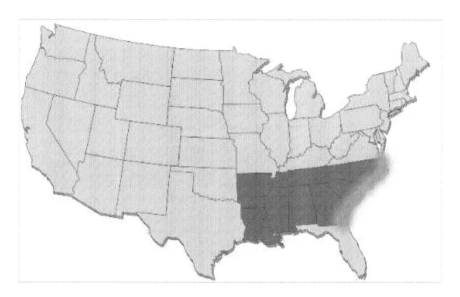

In the U.S., stroke mortality is unusually high in a cluster of Southeastern states known as the Stroke Belt. In the Belt's "buckle" (edge), stroke mortality may be double the national average.

Several decades ago, scientists and statisticians noticed that people in the southeastern United States had the highest stroke mortality rate in the country. They named this region the **stroke belt**. For many years, researchers believed that the increased risk was due to the higher percentage of African-Americans and an overall lower socioeconomic status (SES) in the southern states. A low SES is associated with an overall lower standard of living, leading to a lower standard of health care and therefore an increased risk of stroke. But researchers now know that the higher percentage of African-Americans and the overall lower SES in the southern states does not adequately account for the higher incidence of, and mortality from, stroke in those states. This means that other factors must be contributing to the higher incidence of and mortality from stroke in this region. *(Learn more by end of this textbook)*

Recent studies have also shown that there is a **stroke buckle** in the stroke belt. Three southeastern states, *North Carolina, South Carolina,* and *Georgia,* have an extremely high stroke mortality rate, higher than the rate in other stroke belt states and up to two times the stroke mortality rate of the United States overall. The increased risk could be due to geographic or environmental factors or to regional differences in lifestyle, including higher rates of cigarette smoking and a regional preference for salty, high-fat foods.

Other Risk Factors

The most important risk factors for stroke are hypertension, heart disease, diabetes, and cigarette smoking. Others include heavy alcohol consumption, high blood cholesterol levels, illicit drug use, and genetic or congenital conditions, particularly vascular abnormalities. People with more than one risk factor have what is called "amplification of risk." This means that the multiple risk factors compound their destructive effects and create an overall risk greater than the simple cumulative effect of the individual risk factors.

Hypertension

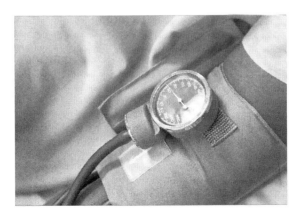

51

Of all the risk factors that contribute to stroke, the most powerful is hypertension, or high blood pressure. People with hypertension have a risk for stroke that is four to six times higher than the risk for those without hypertension. One-third of the adult U.S. population, about 50 million people (including 40-70 percent of those over age 65) have high blood pressure. Forty to 90 percent of stroke patients have high blood pressure before their stroke event.

A systolic pressure of 120 mm of Hg over a diastolic pressure of 80 mm of Hg is generally considered normal. Persistently high **blood pressure greater than 140 over 90** leads to the diagnosis of the disease called hypertension. The impact of hypertension on the total risk for stroke decreases with increasing age, therefore factors other than hypertension play a greater role in the overall stroke risk in elderly adults. For people without hypertension, the absolute risk of stroke increases over time until around the age of 90, when the absolute risk becomes the same as that for people with hypertension.

Like stroke, there is a gender difference in the prevalence of hypertension. In younger people, hypertension is more common among men than among women. With increasing age, however, more women than men have hypertension. This hypertension gender-age difference probably has an impact on the incidence and prevalence of stroke in these populations.

Antihypertensive medication can decrease a person's risk for stroke. Recent studies suggest that treatment can decrease the stroke incidence rate by 38 percent and decrease the stroke fatality rate by 40 percent. Common hypertensive agents include adrenergic agents, beta-blockers, angiotensin converting enzyme inhibitors, calcium channel blockers, diuretics, and vasodilators.

Heart Disease

After hypertension, the second most powerful risk factor for stroke is heart disease, especially a condition known as **atrial fibrillation**. Atrial fibrillation is irregular beating of the left atrium, or left upper chamber, of the heart. In people with atrial fibrillation, the left atrium beats up to four times faster than the rest of the heart. This leads to an irregular flow of blood and the occasional formation of blood clots that can leave the heart and travel to the brain, causing a stroke.

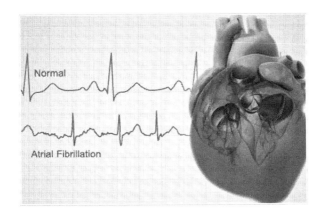

Atrial fibrillation, which affects as many as 2.2 million Americans, increases an individual's risk of stroke by 4 to 6 percent, and about 15 percent of stroke patients have atrial fibrillation before they experience a stroke. The condition is more prevalent in the upper age groups, which means that the prevalence of atrial fibrillation in the United States will increase proportionately with the growth of the elderly population. Unlike hypertension and other risk factors that have a lesser impact on the ever-rising absolute risk of stroke that comes with advancing age, the influence of atrial fibrillation on total risk for stroke increases powerfully with age. In people over 80 years old, atrial fibrillation is the direct cause of one in four strokes.

Other forms of heart disease that increase stroke risk include malformations of the heart valves or the heart muscle. Some valve diseases, like *mitral valve stenosis* or *mitral annular calcification*, can double the risk for stroke, independent of other risk factors.

Heart muscle malformations can also increase the risk for stroke. Patent foramen ovale (PFO) is a passage or a hole (sometimes called a "shunt") in the heart wall separating the two atria, or upper chambers, of the heart. Clots in the blood are usually filtered out by the lungs, but PFO could allow emboli or blood clots to bypass the lungs and go directly through the arteries to the brain, potentially causing a stroke. Research is currently under way to determine how important PFO is as a cause for stroke. Atrial septal aneurysm (ASA), a congenital (present from birth) malformation of the heart tissue, is a bulging of the septum or heart wall into one of the atria of the heart. Researchers do not know why this malformation increases the risk for stroke. PFO and ASA frequently occur together and therefore amplify the risk for stroke. Two other heart malformations that seem to increase the risk for stroke for unknown reasons are left atrial enlargement and left ventricular hypertrophy. People with left atrial enlargement have a larger than normal left atrium of the heart; those with left ventricular hypertrophy have a thickening of the wall of the left ventricle.

Another risk factor for stroke is cardiac surgery to correct heart malformations or reverse the effects of heart disease. Strokes occurring in this situation are usually the result of surgically dislodged plaques from the aorta that travel through the bloodstream to the arteries in the neck and head, causing stroke. Cardiac surgery increases a person's risk of stroke by about 1 percent. Other types of surgery can also increase the risk of stroke.

Blood Cholesterol Levels

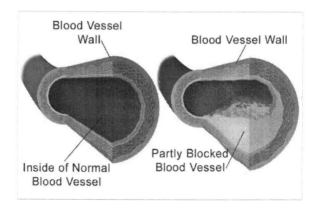

Most people know that **high cholesterol levels** contribute to heart disease. But many don't realize that a high cholesterol level also contributes to stroke risk. Cholesterol, a waxy substance produced by the liver, is a vital body product. It contributes to the production of hormones and vitamin D and is an integral component of cell membranes. The liver makes enough cholesterol to fuel the body's needs and this natural production of cholesterol alone is not a large contributing factor to atherosclerosis, heart disease, and stroke. Research has shown that the danger from cholesterol comes from a dietary intake of foods that contain high levels of cholesterol. Foods high in saturated fat and cholesterol, like meats, eggs, and dairy products, can increase the amount of total cholesterol in the body to alarming levels, contributing to the risk of atherosclerosis and thickening of the arteries.

Cholesterol is classified as a lipid, meaning that it is fat-soluble rather than water-soluble. Other lipids include fatty acids, glycerides, alcohol, waxes, steroids, and fat-soluble vitamins A, D, and E. Lipids and water, like oil and water, do not mix. Blood is a water-based liquid, therefore cholesterol does not mix with blood. In order to travel through the blood without clumping together, cholesterol needs to be covered by a layer of protein. The cholesterol and protein together are called a *lipoprotein*.

There are two kinds of cholesterol, commonly called the "good" and the "bad." Good cholesterol is *high-density lipoprotein*, or *HDL*; bad cholesterol is *low-density lipoprotein*, or *LDL*. Together, these two forms of cholesterol make up a person's *total serum cholesterol* level. Most cholesterol tests measure the level of total cholesterol in the blood and don't distinguish between good and bad cholesterol. For these total serum cholesterol tests, a level of less than 200 mg/dL is considered safe, while a level of more than 240 is considered dangerous and places a person at risk for heart disease and stroke.

Most cholesterol in the body is in the form of LDL. LDLs circulate through the bloodstream, picking up excess cholesterol and depositing cholesterol where it is needed (for example, for the production and maintenance of cell membranes). But when too much cholesterol starts circulating in the blood, the body cannot handle the excessive LDLs, which build up along the inside of the arterial walls. The buildup of LDL coating on the inside of the artery walls hardens and turns into arterial plaque, leading to stenosis and atherosclerosis. This plaque blocks blood vessels and contributes to the formation of blood clots. A person's LDL level should be less than 130 mg/dL to be safe. LDL levels between 130 and 159 put a person at a slightly higher risk for atherosclerosis, heart disease, and stroke. A score over 160 puts a person at great risk for a heart attack or stroke.

The other form of cholesterol, HDL, is beneficial and contributes to stroke prevention. HDL carries a small percentage of the cholesterol in the blood, but instead of depositing its cholesterol on the inside of artery walls, HDL returns to the liver to unload its cholesterol. The liver then eliminates the excess cholesterol by passing it along to the kidneys. Currently, any HDL score higher than 35 is considered desirable. Recent studies have shown that high levels of HDL are associated with a reduced risk for heart disease and stroke and that low levels (less than 35 mg/dL), even in people with normal levels of LDL, lead to an increased risk for heart disease and stroke.

A person may lower his risk for atherosclerosis and stroke by improving his cholesterol levels. A healthy diet and regular exercise are the best ways to lower total cholesterol levels. In some cases, physicians may prescribe cholesterol-lowering medication, and recent studies have shown that the newest types of these drugs, called reductase inhibitors or statin drugs, significantly reduce the risk for stroke in most patients with high cholesterol. Scientists believe that statins may work by reducing the amount of bad cholesterol the body produces and by reducing the body's inflammatory immune reaction to cholesterol plaque associated with atherosclerosis and stroke.

* mm of Hg-or millimeters of mercury-is the standard means of expressing blood pressure, which is measured using an instrument called a sphygmomanometer. Using a stethoscope and a cuff that is wrapped around the patient's upper arm, a health professional listens

to the sounds of blood rushing through an artery. The first sound registered on the instrument gauge (which measures the pressure of the blood in millimeters on a column of mercury) is called the systolic pressure. This is the maximum pressure produced as the left ventricle of the heart contracts and the blood begins to flow through the artery. The second sound is the diastolic pressure and is the lowest pressure in the artery when the left ventricle is relaxing.

** mg/dL describes the weight of cholesterol in milligrams in a deciliter of blood. This is the standard way of measuring blood cholesterol levels.

Diabetes

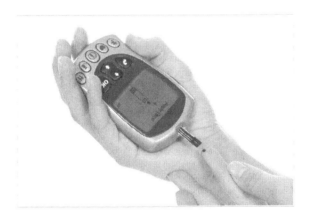

Diabetes is another disease that increases a person's risk for stroke. People with diabetes have three times the risk of stroke compared to people without diabetes. The relative risk of stroke from diabetes is highest in the fifth and sixth decades of life and decreases after that. Like hypertension, the relative risk of stroke from diabetes is highest for men at an earlier age and highest for women at an older age. People with diabetes may also have other contributing risk factors that can amplify the overall risk for stroke. For example, the prevalence of hypertension is 40 percent higher in the diabetic population compared to the general population.

DERBY PUBLIC LIBRARY

Sickle Cell Disease

Sickle cell disease is a blood disorder associated with ischemic stroke that mainly affects black and Hispanic children. The disease causes some red blood cells to form an abnormal sickle shape. A stroke can happen if sickle cells get stuck in a blood vessel and block the flow of blood to the brain.

Modifiable Lifestyle Risk Factors

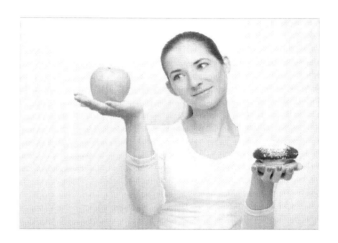

Unhealthy Diet. Diets high in saturated fats, trans fat, and cholesterol have been linked to stroke and related conditions, such as heart disease. Also, too much salt (sodium) in the diet can raise blood pressure levels.

Physical Inactivity. Not getting enough physical activity can increase the chances of having other risk factors for stroke, including obesity, high blood pressure, high cholesterol, and diabetes. Regular physical activity can lower your risk for stroke.

Obesity. Obesity is excess body fat. Obesity is linked to higher "bad" cholesterol and triglyceride levels and to lower "good" cholesterol levels. In addition to heart disease, obesity can also lead to high blood pressure and diabetes.

Cigarette smoking. Cigarette smoking is the most powerful modifiable stroke risk factor. Smoking almost doubles a person's risk for ischemic stroke, independent of other risk factors, and it increases a person's risk for subarachnoid hemorrhage by up to 3.5 percent. Smoking is directly responsible for a greater percentage of the total number of strokes in young adults than in older adults. Risk factors other than smoking - like hypertension, heart disease, and diabetes - account for more of the total number of strokes in older adults.

Heavy smokers are at greater risk for stroke than light smokers. The relative risk of stroke decreases immediately after quitting smoking, with a major reduction of risk seen after 2 to 4 years. Unfortunately, it may take several decades for a former smoker's risk to drop to the level of someone who never smoked.

Smoking increases the risk of stroke by promoting atherosclerosis and increasing the levels of blood-clotting factors, such as fibrinogen. In addition to promoting conditions linked to stroke, smoking also increases the damage that results from stroke by weakening the *endothelial wall* of the cerebrovascular system. This leads to greater damage to the brain from events that occur in the secondary stage of stroke.

High alcohol consumption. High alcohol consumption is another modifiable risk factor for stroke. Generally, an increase in alcohol consumption leads to an increase in blood pressure. While scientists agree that heavy drinking is a risk for both hemorrhagic and ischemic stroke, in several research studies daily consumption of smaller amounts of alcohol has been found to provide a protective influence against ischemic stroke, perhaps because alcohol decreases the clotting ability of *platelets* in the blood. Moderate alcohol consumption may act in the same way as aspirin to decrease blood clotting and prevent ischemic stroke. Heavy alcohol consumption, though, may seriously deplete platelet numbers and compromise blood clotting and blood viscosity, leading to hemorrhage. In addition, heavy drinking or binge drinking can lead to a rebound effect after the alcohol is purged from the body. The consequences of this rebound effect are that blood viscosity (thickness) and platelet levels skyrocket after heavy drinking, increasing the risk for ischemic stroke.

Illicit drugs. The use of illicit drugs, such as cocaine and crack cocaine, can cause stroke. Cocaine may act on other risk factors, such as hypertension, heart disease, and vascular disease, to trigger a stroke. It decreases relative cerebrovascular blood flow by up to 30 percent, causes vascular constriction, and inhibits vascular relaxation, leading to narrowing of the arteries. Cocaine also affects the heart, causing arrhythmias and rapid heart rate that can lead to the formation of blood clots.

Marijuana smoking. Marijuana smoking may also be a risk factor for stroke. Marijuana decreases blood pressure and may interact with other risk factors, such as hypertension and cigarette smoking, to cause rapidly fluctuating blood pressure levels, damaging blood vessels.

Drugs abuse. Other drugs abuse, such as amphetamines, heroin, and anabolic steroids (and even some common, legal drugs, such as caffeine and L-asparaginase and pseudoephedrine found in over-the-counter decongestants), have been suspected of increasing stroke risk. Many of these drugs are vasoconstrictors, meaning that they cause blood vessels to constrict and blood pressure to rise.

Head and Neck Injuries

Injuries to the head or neck may damage the cerebrovascular system and cause a small number of strokes. Head injury or traumatic brain injury may cause bleeding within the brain leading to damage akin to that caused by a hemorrhagic stroke. Neck injury, when associated with spontaneous tearing of the vertebral or carotid arteries caused by sudden and severe extension of the neck, neck rotation, or pressure on the artery, is a contributing cause of stroke, especially in young adults. This type of stroke is often called "beauty-parlor syndrome," which refers to the practice of extending the neck backwards over a sink for hair-washing in beauty parlors. Neck calisthenics, "bottoms-up" drinking, and improperly performed chiropractic manipulation of the neck can also put strain on the vertebral and carotid arteries, possibly leading to ischemic stroke.

Infections

Recent viral and bacterial infections may act with other risk factors to add a small risk for stroke. The immune system responds to infection by increasing inflammation and increasing the infection-fighting properties of the blood. Unfortunately, this immune response increases the number of clotting factors in the blood, leading to an increased risk of embolic-ischemic stroke.

Genetic Risk Factors

Although there may not be a single genetic factor associated with stroke, genes do play a large role in the expression of stroke risk factors such as hypertension, heart disease, diabetes, and vascular malformations. It is also possible that an increased risk for stroke within a family is due to environmental factors, such as a common sedentary lifestyle or poor eating habits, rather than hereditary factors.

Vascular malformations that cause stroke may have the strongest genetic link of all stroke risk factors. A vascular malformation is an abnormally formed blood vessel or group of blood vessels. One genetic vascular disease called CADASIL, which stands for cerebral autosomal dominant arteriopathy with subcortical infarcts and leukoencephalopathy. CADASIL is a rare, genetically inherited, congenital vascular disease of the brain that causes strokes, subcortical dementia, migraine-like headaches, and psychiatric disturbances. CADASIL is very debilitating and symptoms usually surface around the age of 45. Although CADASIL can be treated with surgery to repair the defective blood vessels, patients often die by the age of 65. The exact incidence of CADASIL in the United States is unknown.

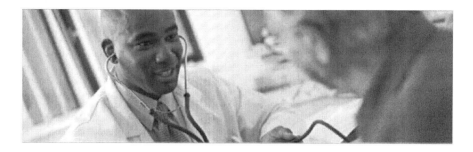

If you have heart disease, high cholesterol, high blood pressure, or diabetes you can take steps to lower your risk for stroke.

Check Cholesterol

Your health care provider should test your cholesterol levels at least once every 5 years. Talk with your health care team about this simple blood test. If you have high cholesterol, medications and lifestyle changes can help reduce your risk for stroke.

Control Blood Pressure

High blood pressure usually has no symptoms, so be sure to have it checked on a regular basis. Talk to your health care team about how often you should check your levels. You can check your blood pressure at home, at a doctor's office, or at a pharmacy.

If you have high blood pressure, your doctor might prescribe medication, recommend some changes in your lifestyle, or advise you to lower the levels of salt in your diet.

Manage Diabetes

If your health care provider thinks you have symptoms of diabetes, he or she may recommend that you get tested. If you have diabetes, monitor your blood sugar levels carefully. Talk with your health care team about treatment options. Your doctor may recommend certain lifestyle changes to help keep your blood sugar under good control—those actions will help reduce your risk for stroke.

Manage Heart Disease

If you have certain heart conditions such as atrial fibrillation (irregular heartbeat), your health care team may recommend medical treatment or surgery. Taking care of heart problems can help prevent stroke.

Take Your Medicine

If you take medication to treat heart disease, high cholesterol, high blood pressure, or diabetes, follow your doctor's instructions carefully. Always ask questions if you don't understand something. Never stop taking your medication without talking to your doctor or pharmacist.

Talk with Your Health Care Team

You and your health care team can work together to prevent or treat the medical conditions that lead to stroke. Discuss your treatment plan regularly, and bring a list of questions to your appointments.

If you've already had a stroke or TIA, your health care team will work with you to prevent further strokes. Your treatment plan will include medications or surgery and lifestyle changes to reduce your risk for another stroke. Be sure to take your medications as directed and follow your doctor's instructions.

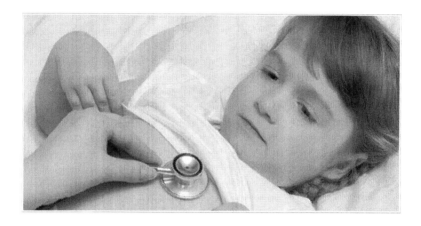

Compared to stroke in the adult brain, stroke in the young, growing brain is associated with unique symptoms, risk factors, and outcomes - and with more uncertainty in all three of these areas. Although stroke is often considered a disease of aging, the risk of stroke in childhood is actually highest during the perinatal period, which encompasses the last few months of fetal life and the first few weeks after birth.

As in adults, the symptoms of stroke in infants and children include headache, hemiplegia, and hemiparesis. But very young children with stroke are more likely than adults to experience other symptoms, such as seizures, breathing problems, or loss of consciousness. Because the incidence of childhood stroke is relatively low, parents and doctors often mistakenly attribute these symptoms to other causes, leading to delays in diagnosis. Moreover, the time of onset is usually unknown for strokes during the perinatal period.

Investigators know less about the risk of childhood stroke than they know about the risk of adult stroke. However, well-documented risk factors include congenital (inborn) heart abnormalities, head trauma, and blood-clotting disorders. An important risk factor for African American children is sickle cell disease. Although sickle

64

cell disease is known for its effect on red blood cells - causing them to take on a sickle shape - it can also cause a narrowing of cerebral arteries. A 1998 study of some 3,000 people with sickle cell disease found that 11 percent experienced a stroke before age 20. Fortunately, that same year, a study funded by NHLBI showed that repeated transfusions to replace sickled blood cells with normal blood cells reduced the risk of stroke by 92 percent. Yearly Doppler ultrasound imaging is recommended for young children with sickle cell disease and, if stenosis is found, repeated transfusions can be used as a means of stroke prevention.

Strokes during the perinatal period have been associated with premature birth, maternal infections, maternal drug abuse, prior infertility treatments, and maternal health conditions such as autoimmune disease and preeclampsia (a potentially serious combination of hypertension and kidney problems that affects about six percent of pregnant women).

The outcome of stroke in the very young is difficult to predict. A stroke during fetal development may lead to cerebral palsy - a permanent problem with body movement and muscle coordination that appears in infancy or early childhood. A stroke that occurs during infancy or childhood can also cause permanent disability. Generally, outcomes are worse in children under age one and in those who experience decreased consciousness or seizures. Fortunately, the developing brain is also known for its remarkable capacity to replace lost nerve cells and fix damaged connections between them. Healthy areas of the brain are often still pliable enough to compensate for damaged areas.

A child with serious deficits immediately after a stroke can make an impressive recovery.

Treatment of stroke in children presents unique challenges. Delays in diagnosis, which can be especially prolonged in cases of perinatal stroke, mean that valuable time is lost. Moreover, most treatments for acute stroke were developed based on studies in adults and the guidelines for their use in children are still being refined. To address some of these issues, NINDS and NIH's

National Institute of Child Health and Human Development (NICHD) sponsored a workshop on perinatal stroke in August 2006 that brought together experts in pediatrics, neurology, cardiology, and public health. Goals set by this group include the development and testing of new therapies for perinatal stroke, a better understanding of the risk factors for it, and improved brain imaging methods to diagnose it.

From ages 55 to 75, the annual incidence and short-term risk of stroke are higher in men than in women. However, because women generally live longer than men, their lifetime risk of stroke is higher and they account for a larger fraction (about 61 percent) of stroke deaths each year.

Women have unique stroke risks associated with **pregnancy** and **menopause**. In women of childbearing age, the risk of stroke is relatively low (with an annual incidence of one in 10,000), but a recent study estimates that pregnancy increases that risk three-fold.

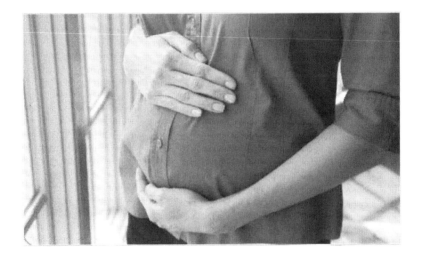

Several factors contribute to the increased risk of stroke during pregnancy. The activity of blood clotting proteins is naturally amplified during pregnancy, increasing the chances of ischemic stroke for the mother (and perhaps contributing to perinatal stroke). Most maternal strokes occur during the first several weeks after delivery, suggesting that the drop in blood volume or the rapid hormonal changes following childbirth also play a role. Pregnancy-related stroke is more likely to occur in women who experience certain complications, such as infections or preeclampsia, or who have other risk factors for stroke, such as hypertension or diabetes.

Hormone replacement therapy (HRT) may ease the discomfort and the loss of bone density associated with menopause. It was once considered a possible means of stroke prevention in post-menopausal women. However, a series of placebo-controlled clinical trials sponsored by NINDS and NHLBI has shown that HRT increases the risk of stroke. NHLBI's Women's Health Initiative showed that treatment with the hormones estrogen and progestin increased the risk of stroke by 31 percent in women with an intact uterus. In women who had undergone a hysterectomy, treatment with estrogen alone increased the risk of stroke by 39 percent. The NINDS Women's Estrogen for Stroke Trial (WEST) found that women who had experienced a prior ischemic stroke and received estrogen were more likely to have a fatal recurrent stroke.

PREVENTION OF STROKE

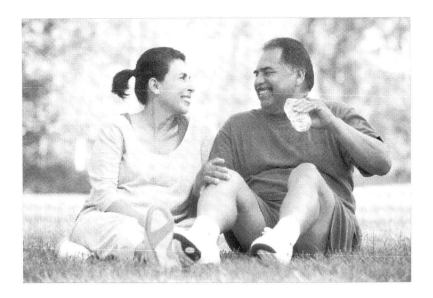

You can help prevent stroke by making healthy lifestyle choices. A healthy lifestyle includes the following:

- Eating a healthy diet.
- Maintaining a healthy weight.
- Getting enough exercise.
- Not smoking.
- Limiting alcohol use.
- Combination Therapies.

Healthy Diet

Choosing healthy meal and snack options can help you avoid stroke and its complications. Be sure to eat plenty of fresh fruits and vegetables.

Eating foods low in saturated fats, trans fat, and cholesterol and high in fiber can help prevent high cholesterol. Limiting salt (sodium) in your diet also can lower your blood pressure.

Healthy Weight

Being overweight or obese increases your risk for stroke. To determine whether your weight is in a healthy range, doctors often calculate your body mass index (BMI). Doctors sometimes also use waist and hip measurements to measure excess body fat.

Physical Activity

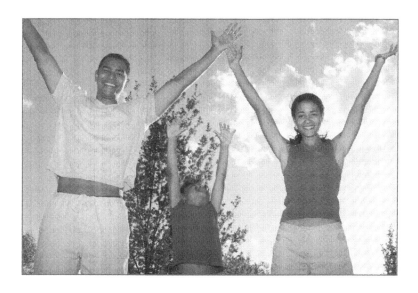

Physical activity can help you maintain a healthy weight and lower your cholesterol and blood pressure levels. For adults, the Surgeon General recommends 2 hours and 30 minutes of moderate-intensity exercise, like brisk walking or bicycling, every week. Children and adolescents should get 1 hour of physical activity every day.

No Smoking

Cigarette smoking greatly increases your risk for stroke. If you don't smoke, don't start. If you do smoke, quitting will lower your risk for stroke. Your doctor can suggest ways to help you quit.

Limited Alcohol

Avoid drinking too much alcohol, which can raise your blood pressure. Men should have no more than 2 drinks per day, and women only 1.

Combination Therapies for Stroke Prevention

Many people at risk for stroke take multiple preventative medications, including antiplatelet drugs, ACE inhibitors, and/or statins. In 2006, NINDS-supported researchers completed the first study to explore whether using these three drugs in combination is more beneficial than using just one or two of them. The researchers examined the medication history and tracked the outcomes of more than 200 individuals who sought care within 24 hours of an ischemic stroke. Individuals taking all three drugs had strokes that were less severe, based on symptoms measured by the NIH Stroke Scale and on MRI scans showing they had less at-risk tissue surrounding the damaged regions of their brains. Individuals on triple therapy also had shorter hospital stays and better function at hospital discharge. Although these data are preliminary, they highlight the possibility of improving stroke outcomes by targeting multiple risk factors.

RESEARCH AND HOPE FOR THE FUTURE

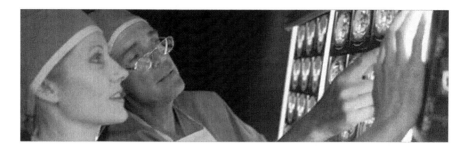

The National Institute of Neurological Disorders and Stroke (NINDS) is the leading supporter of stroke research in the United States and sponsors a wide range of experimental research studies, from investigations of basic **biological mechanisms** to studies with animal models and clinical trials.

Currently, NINDS researchers are studying the mechanisms of stroke risk factors and the process of brain damage that results from stroke. Some of this brain damage may be secondary to the initial death of brain cells caused by the lack of blood flow to the brain tissue. This secondary wave of brain injury is a result of a toxic reaction to the primary damage and mainly involves the excitatory neurochemical, *glutamate*. Glutamate in the normal brain functions as a chemical messenger between brain cells, allowing them to communicate. But an excess amount of glutamate in the brain causes too much activity and brain cells quickly *"burn out"* from too much excitement, releasing more toxic chemicals, such as caspases, cytokines, monocytes, and oxygen-free radicals. These substances poison the chemical environment of surrounding cells, initiating a cascade of degeneration and programmed cell death, called *apoptosis*. NINDS researchers are studying the mechanisms underlying this secondary insult, which consists mainly of inflammation, toxicity, and a breakdown of the blood vessels that provide blood to the brain. Researchers are also looking for ways to prevent secondary injury to the brain by providing different types of neuroprotection for salvagable cells that prevent inflammation and block some of the toxic chemicals created by dying brain cells.

From this research, scientists hope to develop neuroprotective agents to prevent secondary damage.

Basic research has also focused on the genetics of stroke and stroke risk factors. One area of research involving genetics is **gene therapy**. Gene therapy involves putting a gene for a desired protein in certain cells of the body. The inserted gene will then "program" the cell to produce the desired protein. If enough cells in the right areas produce enough protein, then the protein could be therapeutic. Scientists must find ways to deliver the therapeutic DNA to the appropriate cells and must learn how to deliver enough DNA to enough cells so that the tissues produce a therapeutic amount of protein. Gene therapy is in the very early stages of development and there are many problems to overcome, including learning how to penetrate the highly impermeable *blood-brain barrier* and how to halt the host's immune reaction to the virus that carries the gene to the cells. Some of the proteins used for stroke therapy could include neuroprotective proteins, anti-inflammatory proteins, and DNA/cellular repair proteins, among others.

The NINDS supports and conducts a wide variety of studies in **animals**, from genetics research on zebrafish to rehabilitation research on primates. Much of the Institute's animal research involves rodents, specifically mice and rats. For example, one study of hypertension and stroke uses rats that have been bred to be hypertensive and therefore stroke-prone. By studying stroke in rats, scientists hope to get a better picture of what might be happening in human stroke patients. Scientists can also use animal models to test promising therapeutic interventions for stroke. If a therapy proves to be beneficial to animals, then scientists can consider testing the therapy in human subjects.

One promising area of stroke animal research involves **hibernation**. The dramatic decrease of blood flow to the brain in hibernating animals is extensive - extensive enough that it would kill a non-hibernating animal. During hibernation, an animal's metabolism slows down, body temperature drops, and energy and oxygen requirements of brain cells decrease. If scientists can discover how animals hibernate without experiencing brain damage, then maybe they can discover ways to stop the brain damage associated with decreased blood flow in stroke patients. Other studies are looking at the role of **hypothermia**, or decreased body temperature, on metabolism and neuroprotection.

Both hibernation and hypothermia have a relationship to *hypoxia* and *edema*. Hypoxia, or *anoxia*, occurs when there is not enough oxygen available for brain cells to function properly. Since brain cells require large amounts of oxygen for energy requirements, they are especially vulnerable to hypoxia. Edema occurs when the chemical balance of brain tissue is disturbed and water or fluids flow into the brain cells, making them swell and burst, releasing their toxic contents into the surrounding tissues. Edema is one cause of general brain tissue swelling and contributes to the secondary injury associated with stroke.

The basic and animal studies discussed above do not involve people and fall under the category of preclinical research; clinical research involves people. One area of investigation that has made the transition from animal models to clinical research is the study of the mechanisms underlying brain plasticity and the neuronal rewiring that occurs after a stroke.

New advances in imaging and rehabilitation have shown that the brain can compensate for function lost as a result of stroke. When cells in an area of the brain responsible for a particular function die after a stroke, the patient becomes unable to perform that function. For example, a stroke patient with an infarct in the area of the brain responsible for facial recognition becomes unable to recognize faces, a syndrome called facial *agnosia*. But, in time, the person may come to recognize faces again, even though the area of the brain originally programmed to perform that function remains dead. The plasticity of the brain and the rewiring of the neural connections make it possible for one part of the brain to change functions and take up the more important functions of a disabled part. This **rewiring** of the brain and **restoration** of function, which the brain tries to do automatically, can be helped with therapy. Scientists are working to develop new and better ways to help the brain repair itself to restore important functions to the stroke patient.

One example of a therapy resulting from this research is the use of **transcranial magnetic stimulation (TMS)** in stroke rehabilitation. Some evidence suggests that TMS, in which a small magnetic current is delivered to an area of the brain, may possibly increase brain plasticity and speed up recovery of function after a stroke. The TMS device is a small coil which is held outside of the head, over the part of the brain needing stimulation. Currently, several studies at the NINDS are testing whether TMS has any value in increasing motor function and improving functional recovery.

FINDINGS FROM RECENTLY COMPLETED CLINICAL TRIALS

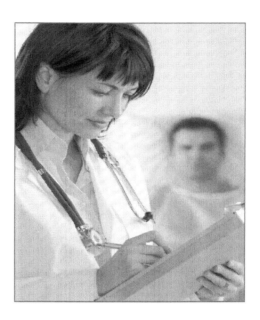

NINDS conducts clinical trials at the NIH Clinical Center and also provides funding for clinical trials at hospitals and universities across the United States and Canada. Below are findings from some of the largest and most significant recent clinical trials in stroke, as well as summaries of some of the most promising clinical trials in progress.

Warfarin versus Aspirin for Intracranial Arterial Stenosis

The goal of this trial was to compare the effectiveness of warfarin to aspirin in preventing subsequent strokes or other vascular-related events, such as heart attacks, in people with clogged arteries in the brain (intracranial arterial stenosis). It was ended early when **aspirin was shown to be clearly superior to warfarin** in preventing subsequent strokes. Aspirin also causes fewer and less serious side effects, costs less, and is easier to use.

Extremity Constraint-Induced Therapy Evaluation

Impaired movement in the arms and legs is a major consequence of stroke. Methods to improve motor function and return the independent use of arms and hands are limited. One technique that had been shown to be successful in basic research studies with animal and human subjects was **constraint-induced movement therapy (CIMT)**. CIMT involves restriction of the stronger arm, while the weaker arm is put through a series of repetitive exercises. The trial randomly sorted stroke patients who had had a stroke within the past 3 to 9 months and who had at least minimal ability in their arms into two groups - one that received customary care (which ranged from no treatment to standard physical therapy) and one that received CIMT. CIMT involved training for several hours, every weekday, for 2 weeks. Participants in both groups of the trial were tested immediately after treatment, and then 4, 8, and 12 months later with a series of tasks designed to measure arm dexterity. They were also asked to report how often they used the weaker arm in daily activities. Overall, the participants in the CIMT group showed significantly improved function in the weaker arm at each time tested, even almost a year after the training had ended.

The Carotid Revascularization Endarterectomy vs. Stenting Trial

The use of dilation and stenting techniques similar to those used to unclog and open heart arteries has been proposed as a less invasive alternative to carotid endarterectomy (surgery to remove the buildup of plaque within the carotid artery, which supplies blood to the head and neck). Carotid endarterectomy is considered the gold standard treatment for preventing stroke and other vascular events. Stenting is a newer, less invasive procedure in which an expandable metal stent (tube) is inserted into the carotid artery to keep it open after it has been widened with balloon dilation. The study showed that the **overall safety and effectiveness of the two procedures was largely the same**—with equal benefits for both men and women, and for people who had previously had a stroke and for those who had not. Physicians will now have more options to tailor treatments for people at risk for stroke.

Carotid Occlusion Surgery Study

The goal of this randomized clinical trial was to determine the preventive power of extracranial bypass surgery in a group of stroke survivors who have both a blocked carotid artery and an increased oxygen extraction fraction (or OEF, which indicates how hard the brain has to work to pull oxygen from the blood supply). An increased OEF has been shown to be a powerful and independent risk factor for subsequent stroke. Extracranial bypass surgery uses a healthy blood vessel to detour blood flow around the site of the blocked artery and results in increased blood flow to the brain. The results showed that in spite of the surgical success of improving cerebral blood flow, **extracranial-intracranial bypass surgery did not demonstrate any benefit** in reducing the risk of having a stroke recurrence due to the much better than expected recurrence rate in the non-surgical medical alone group.

Locomotor Experience Applied Post-Stroke

Only 37 percent of stroke survivors are able to walk after the first week following their stroke. The investigators of the Locomotor Experience Applied Post-Stroke (LEAPS) trial set out to compare the effectiveness of the body-weight supported treadmill training with walking practice started at two different stages--two months post-stroke (early locomotor training) and six months post-stroke (late locomotor training). The locomotor training was also compared against a home exercise program managed by a physical therapist, aimed at enhancing patients' flexibility, range of motion, strength and balance as a way to improve their walking. The primary measure was each group's improvement in walking at one year after the stroke. The study found that stroke patients who had **physical therapy at home improved their ability to walk just as well as those who were treated in a training program** that requires the use of a body-weight supported treadmill device followed by

78

walking practice. In addition, the study also found that patients continued to improve up to one year after stroke, defying conventional wisdom that recovery occurs early and tops out at six months.

Secondary Prevention of Small Subcortical Strokes

In this trial, investigators are testing new approaches to stroke prevention for people with a history of small subcortical strokes. The trial was designed to compare: 1) aspirin alone vs. combined antiplatelet therapy (aspirin and clopidogrel), and 2) intensive vs. standard blood pressure control. Subcortical strokes, also called lacunar strokes, occur when the thread-like arteries within cerebral tissue become blocked and halt blood flow to the brain. They account for up to one-fifth of all strokes in the U.S. and are especially common among people of Hispanic descent. In the antiplatelet component of SPS3, researchers have found that the **combined antiplatelet therapy was about equal to aspirin** in reducing stroke risk, but it almost doubled the risk of gastrointestinal bleeding. The blood pressure component of the trial is ongoing.

Stenting vs. Aggressive Medical Management for Preventing Recurrent Stroke in Intracranial Stenosis

The best treatment for preventing another stroke or TIA in patients with narrowing of a brain artery is uncertain. The purpose of this trial was to compare the safety and effectiveness of aggressive medical treatment (i.e., intensive management of key stroke risk factors including blood pressure, cholesterol, and lifestyle modification) alone to aggressive medical therapy plus a Food and Drug Administration (FDA)-approved intracranial stent to prevent another stroke in individuals who recently had either a transient ischemic attack or non-disabling stroke. The results of this trial, which was stopped early, showed that the group that received the **intensive medical management alone had better outcomes than the group who also received the stent**. This study provides an answer to a long-standing question by physicians—what to do to prevent a devastating second stroke in a high risk population.

TEENAGE YEARS IN "STROKE BELT" DRIVE UP RISK

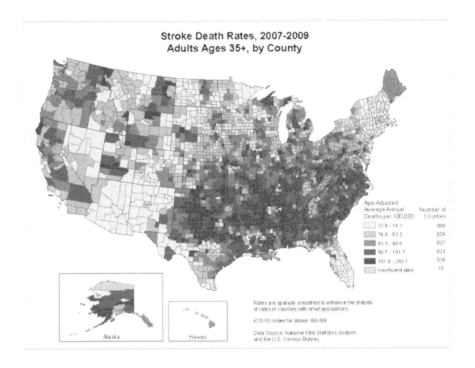

Stroke Death Rates, 2007-2009
Adults Ages 35+, by County

Adolescence is inarguably a vulnerable time of life, but a new study suggests that spending it living in the **southeastern United States region** known as the *"Stroke Belt"* adds an extra hazard: It raises one's risk of stroke later in life.

In a large population-based study funded by the National Institute of Neurological Disorders and Stroke (NINDS), people who spent their teenage years (ages 13-18) living in the Stroke Belt had a **17% higher risk of stroke** than those who spent no time living in the region.

The magnitude of harm from Stroke Belt living was greater among **blacks** than among whites. Compared to study volunteers who spent no time living in the Stroke Belt, a lifetime in the region increased stroke risk by 35% among blacks and by 15% among whites. Blacks who spent only their adolescence in the Stroke Belt were at 33% greater risk; whites had a 15% higher risk.

Researchers followed 24,544 black and white people of a mean age of 65 and who were stroke-free at the start of the study. During the next six years, 615 study participants suffered their first stroke.

Adolescence is a malleable period during which unhealthy lifestyle choices get established, said the study's lead investigator Virginia J. Howard, Ph.D., of the University of Alabama at Birmingham. People who smoke, for example, often start during their teenage years. At the same time, "areas of the Southeast have been shown to have among the lowest levels of healthy behaviors such as regular physical activity and the highest prevalence of cardiovascular factors, such as hypertension and obesity," she wrote.

BIBLIOGRAPHY

Centers for Disease Control and Prevention. *Stroke.* Retrieved April 16, 2014 from http://www.cdc.gov/stroke/

National Institute of Neurological Disorders and Stroke. National Institute of Health. *NINDS Stroke Information Page.* Retrieved April 16, 2014 from http://www.ninds.nih.gov/disorders/stroke/stroke.htm

National Institute of Neurological Disorders and Stroke. National Institute of Health. *Stroke: Hope Through Research.* Retrieved April 16, 2014 from http://www.ninds.nih.gov/disorders/stroke/detail_stroke.htm

National Institute of Neurological Disorders and Stroke. National Institute of Health. *NIH-funded study suggests that moving more may lower stroke risk.* Retrieved April 16, 2014 from http://www.ninds.nih.gov/news_and_events/news_articles/pressrelease_stroke_exercise_07182013.htm

National Institute of Neurological Disorders and Stroke. National Institute of Health. *Teenage Years in the "Stroke Belt" Drive up Risk.* Retrieved April 16, 2014 from http://www.ninds.nih.gov/news_and_events/news_articles/stroke_belt_teen_risk.htm

National Institute of Neurological Disorders and Stroke. National Institute of Health. *Landmark NIH Clinical Trial Comparing Two Stroke Prevention Procedures Shows Surgery and Stenting Equally Safe and Effective.* Retrieved April 16, 2014 from http://www.ninds.nih.gov/news_and_events/news_articles/CREST_trial_results_published.htm

Stroke. National Institute of Health. *Know Stroke: Know The Signs. Act In Time.* Retrieved April 16, 2014 from http://stroke.nih.gov/

Stroke. National Institute of Health. *Stroke: Hope Through Research.* Retrieved April 16, 2014 from http://stroke.nih.gov/materials/hopethroughresearch.htm

39381283R00054

Made in the USA
Lexington, KY
20 February 2015